Adverse Cardiovascular Effects of Inactivity Compared to Beneficial Cardiovascular and Sleep Effects of Physical Activity

Adverse Cardiovascular Effects of Inactivity Compared to Beneficial Cardiovascular and Sleep Effects of Physical Activity

Steven G. Chrysant

ELIVA PRESS

ISBN: 978-99949-8-332-2

Cover Design: Eliva Press
Cover Image: Ingimage
Email: info@elivapress.com
Website: www.elivapress.com

This Eliva Press imprint is published by the registered company Eliva Press Global Ltd. part of Eliva Press S.R.L. Publishing Group

The registered company address is: Pope Hennessy Street Level 2, Hennessy Tower Port Louis, Mauritius
Eliva Press S.R.L. Publishing Group address is: Bulevardul Moscova 21, Chisinau, Moldova, Europe

The Adverse Cardiovascular Effects of Inactivity Compared to the Beneficial Cardiovascular and Sleep Effects of Physical Activity in Men and Women

Running Title: Stay Physically Active and Live Better and Longer

Steven G. Chrysant, MD, PhD. Clinical Professor of Medicine University of Oklahoma Health Sciences Center, Oklahoma City, OK

Email: schrysant@yahoo.com

Prologue

We as well as other investigators have previously reported that prolonged sitting time, like watching TV and computer viewing are associated with increased incidence of obesity, type 2 diabetes mellitus (T2DM), cardiovascular disease (CVD), coronary heart disease (CHD), hypertension, and death. In contrast, regular physical activity (PA) of different types and grades is associated with significant reduction of cardiomemetabolic risk, improvement in cardiorespiratory fitness, and overall cardiovascular health, in healthy, as well as in people with preexisting CVD, CHD, T2DM, HF, or frail health. Another major benefit of exercise is its effects on the onset, duration, and quality of sleep. A good sleep quality is essential for physical, cardiovascular and mental health according to American Academy of Sleep Medicine and the Sleep Research Society. For the preparation of this book, a Medline search of the English medical literature was contacted between 2014 and 2023. The data from this search of literature in combination with collateral literature will be discussed in this book.

Contents

Chapter One

Adverse Cardiovascular Effects of Inactivity and Excessive Sitting Time

Introduction

The cause of inactivity or excessive sitting time is the result of urbanization and technological advances, which have significantly limited the mobility and increased the sitting time of people at work, at home, and the commute to work. It has been estimated that sitting time occupies about 55% of daily waking time, excluding sleep [1]. There is increasing evidence from prospective studies demonstrating the detrimental effects of excessive sitting time on the incidence of cardiovascular disease (CVD), obesity, type 2 diabetes mellitus (T2DM), and hypertension in the US and other developed countries [3-13]. These studies show that currently, people spend an excessive amount of time sitting in front of computer at work or at home, watching television (TV), playing video games, speaking on the telephone, and commuting to work. The harm of excessive sitting or sedentary behaviors on the cardiometabolic changes and risk of CVD are highlighted in recent publications [13-20], and the data from these studies will be presented in collaboration with other studies.

Studies Demonstrating an Association between Prolonged Sitting Time and Cardiovascular Morbidity and Mortality

Several studies have shown an association of sedentary behavior and increased incidence of CVD and death [4-20]. These studies are summarized in table 1 and they will be, briefly, discussed here. The study by Study by Patel et al [3], is a large prospective study of US adults to examine the leisure time spent on sitting and physical activity (PA) in relation to mortality acquired by questionnaire. This study included 53,440 men ages 63-65 years and 69,776 women ages 61-63 years, free of CVD at baseline. After a mean follow-up of 14 years, 11,307 (20,6%) deaths occurred in men and 7,923 (11.4%) deaths occurred in women. After adjusting for smoking, obesity and other risk factors, sitting > 6 h/day was associated with a significant increase of death, relative risk (RR) 1.17 (95% CI 1.11-1.24) for men and RR 1.34 (95% CI 1.25-1.44) for women compared to < 3 h of sitting. The associations were strongly associated with CVD mortality. The study by Warren et al [4], also, demonstrated an association between sedentary behaviors and increased CVD mortality in men. This study included 7,744 men ages 20-89 years, free of CVD at baseline. Time spent watching TV and riding in a car was assessed and correlated with CVD mortality. After 21 years of follow-up, and adjusting for age, 377 CVD deaths occurred in those who spent > 23 h/wk of combined sedentary time compared to those spent < 11 h/wk ($p < 0.001$). Regardless of sedentary behavior, older individuals with normal weight and normal BP and being physically active, had reduced CVD mortality. In a study by Dunstan et al [5], the association of prolonged TV viewing time with all-cause mortality, CVD morality, cancer, and non CVD mortality was assessed. This study included 8,800 adults ≥ 25 years who participated in the Australian Diabetes, Obesity, and Lifestyle Study (AusDiab). During 6.6 years of follow-up, there were 284 deaths, of which 87 were caused by CVD. After multiple adjustments for CVD risk factors, viewing TV 2-4 h/wk the CVD mortality incidence was increased, HR 1.19 (95% CI 0.72-1.99) for viewing time 2-4 h/wk, where as the HR was1.80 (95% CI 1.04-2.05) for TV viewing ≥ 4 h/wk. For all-cause mortality the HRs were 1.13 (95% CI 0.87-1.36) and HR 1.46 (95% CI 1.04-2.05) for TV viewing 2-4 h/wk and ≥ 4 h/wk, respectively. In another study Wijndaele et al [6], examined the association between TV viewing time and incidence of nonfatal CVD in 12,608 men and women mean age 61.4 ± 9 years, free of CVD at baseline. After a mean follow-up of 6.9 ± 1.9 years and adjusting for CVD risk factors, TV viewing time was associated with CVD mortality in 2620 of 12,608 subjects (20.8%), HR 1.06 (95% CI 1.03-1.08), nonfatal cardiovascular mortality in 2134 of 12,608 (16.9%), HR 106 (95% CI 1.03-1.09), and for CHD in 940 of 12,608 (0.07%), HR 1.08 (95% CI 1.03-1.13). Adjustment for severe CVD risk factors, partially mediated these associations. Similarly, Stamatakis et al [8], assessed the independent relationships of TV viewing time and other screen-based entertainment with all-cause mortality and CV events, in 4512 subjects (1945 men, 2567 women) ≥ 35 years of age, followed for 4.3 years. During the follow-up, there were 215 CVD events and 325 all-cause mortality deaths. After adjustment for CVD risk factors, the HR for all-cause mortality was 1.52 (95% CI 1.06-2.16) and for CVD events was 2.30 (95% CI 1.33-3.96) for ≥ 4 h/d screen viewing time. Adjusting for PA did not appreciably affect the results. In a similar study, Ford et al [8], examined the association between total screen time (TV + computer) with all-cause mortality in 7350 adult subjects ages 44.3-66.9 years, who participated in the National Health and Nutrition Examination Survey (NHANES) and were followed for a median of 5. 8 years. During the follow-up, 542 deaths occurred of which 190 deaths were due to circulatory system complications. After adjusting for age, participants reporting ≥ 5 h/d viewing screen time had a significant increase in all-cause mortality. After progressively adjusting for increasing numbers of covariates, the HR decreased progressively, but still retained its significance. After adjusting for viewing time by age, 12.7% reported < 1 h/d, 16,4% reported 1 h/d, 37.8% 2 h/d, 18.7% 3 h/d, 10.9% 4 h/d, and 13.5% 5 or more hrs/d. In another study, Matthews et al [9] assessed the association of prolonged sitting time and moderate to vigorous PA (MVPA) with mortality in 240,818 adults ages 50 to 71 years of age, who participated in the National Institutes of Health-American Association of Retired Persons (NIH-AARP) Diet and Health Study, free of CVD at baseline. In participants reporting TV viewing time ≥ 7 h/d, the HR was 1.61 (95% CI 1.47-1.76) for all-cause and CVD mortality compared to < 1 h/d. After adjusting for MVPA > 7 h/wk and TV viewing time ≥ 7 h/d, the HRs for all-cause and CVD mortality were 1.47 (95% CI 1.20-1.79) and 2.00 (95% CI 1.33-3.00), respectively. This study showed that prolonged sitting time is associated with significant all-cause and CVD mortality and that MVPA did not alleviate the risks. Similar results were reported in two other studies by the same authors demonstrating the health risks of too much sitting time [10,11]. In other more recent studies the risks of physical inactivity have been demonstrated [2-18]. A prospective study by Shuval et al 12], of 1269 men from the Cooper Longitudinal Study, mean age 46.2 ± 8.9 years examined the adverse cardiometabolic effects of prolonged sedentary time ≥ 9 h/wk vs ≤ 9.9 h/wk. After a mean follow-up of 9.3 ± 7.4 years, there was a significant increase in triglyceride (TG) levels, TG/HDL-C ratio, BMI, waist circumference, and body fat percentage ($p_{for\ trend} < 0.05$). However, the cardiometabolic markers were less pronounced after adjustment for physical fitness. In another study, Kulinski et al [13] assessed the association between cardiorespiratory fitness and sedentary behavior, independently of exercise activity in 2223 patients ages 12 to 49 years from the NHANES 2003-2004 cohort free of heart disease at baseline.

The daily sedentary time was assessed by an accelerometer as counts/min, where as the cardiorespiratory fitness was assessed in METS by a submaximal exercise with a treadmill test. An additional hour of sedentary time was associated with – 0.12 MET (95% CI – 0.02 to – 0.22, $p = 0.03$)) in men and – 0.24 MET (95% CI -0.10 to – 0.38, p < 001) in women. This study showed that sedentary behavior has an adverse effect on physical fitness. Also, the accelerometer showed objectively, that these subjects spent a large part of their daily leisure time staying inactive. Similar findings have been shown by more recent studies. In a review and meta-analysis by Pandey et al [14], of niew prospective cohort studies involving 720,425 participants mean age 54.5 years, analyzed the association of sedentary time with CVD. After a mean follow-up of 11 years, subjects with the highest sedentary time of 12,5 hr/day had an increased incidence of CVD, HR 1.14 (95% CI 1.09-1.19) compared with those with the lowest sedentary time. However, no apparent risk associated with intermediate sedentary time of 7.5 h/d, was found, HR 1.02 (95% CI 0.96-1.08) In continuous analyses, a nonlinear association between sedentary time and incident CVD was found ($p_{nonlinearity} < 0.001$). A higher risk was noted with a sedentary time > 10 h/d, pooled HR 1.08 (95% CI 1.00-1.14). The study by Lansitie et al [15], is a population-based study involving 660 subjects mean age 68.9 years. This study compared the relationship of sedentary time (ST), light physical activity (LPA), and mild to vigorous physical activity (MVPA) on all-cause mortality, and CVD according to 10 year Framingham risk score (FRS). After 6.2 years of follow-up, the data analyzed by a multivariate regression analysis showed that for each 10 min increase in MVPA and LPA were associated with a negative FRS score, β -0.779 (95% CI – 1.186 to – 0.371, p < 0.001) and LPA the β – 0.293 (95% CI –

0.448 to – 0.138, $p < 0.001$). In contrast, prolonged ST was associated with an increase in the FRS score, β 0.290 (95% CI 0.158-0.421, $p < 0.001$). Also, after adjustment for waist circumference, only the ST was associated with a positive FRS score. For each 10 min increase in LPA there was 6.5% decrease in all-cause mortality, HR 0.935 (95% CI 0.884-0.990, $p = 0.020$) and each 10 min increase in ST there was a 5.6% increase in all-cause mortality, HR 1.056 (95% CI 1.007-1.108, $p = 0.025$). This study showed that any level increase in PA and avoidance of ST are associated with a reduced CV risk in older people.

Possible Mechanisms for the Adverse Cardiovascular Effects of Prolonged Sitting

The precise pathophysiologic mechanism (s) by which sedentary behaviors lead to CVD and all-cause mortality is not clear at present. It has been suggested from animal as well as human studies that cardiometabolic changes linked to prolonged sitting time could be responsible for the development of CVD [16,17]. There is evidence that the lipoprotein lipase (LPL) is reduced by 80% to 90% during sitting compared to standing of ambulating [16]. LPL is critical enzyme for the catabolism of TG-rich lipoproteins in the vascular endothelium leading to decreased TG uptake by the nonexercising large muscles and increased levels of plasma TGs, which in combination with low HDL-C, lead to the development of atherosclerosis. Metabolically, excessive sitting time and low energy expenditure lead to obesity, the metabolic syndrome, T2DM, and hypertension, all significant risk factors for CVD [17]. Another important mechanism might be related to a decreased expression of endothelial NO synthase that is caused by decreased local shear stress as a result of lower blood flow in the limbs from the prolonged sitting time [7]. The direct effect of sitting idle is that the work performed by the large skeletal muscles of the legs, back, and trunk required for the upright movements comes to a halt, leading to precipitous fall of LPL activity with the known adverse metabolic consequences. However, at present, we do not know how prolonged sitting impacts the metabolic processes and underlying mechanisms establishing a cause-effect explanation for the findings of observational studies. Recently, hemodynamic studies on the circulatory system have shown that the vascular endothelium responds differently to different types of shear stress [18]. The endothelium reacts to these forces and conveys information via biochemical signals to maintain vascular homeostasis. Unidirectional laminar shear stress stimulates the synthesis of antiatherogenic vasodilatory molecules such as NO and prostacyclin, where as disturbed laminar shear stress stimulates the production of potent proatherogenic substances such as endothelin-1, vascular adhesion molecules and upregulate endothelial-derived ROS, which blunt the endogenous antioxidant mechanisms and their beneficial effects [19]. It has been shown that the prolonged sitting-induced endothelial dysfunction and a decrease in flow-mediated dilation (FMD), a decrease of popliteal blood flow attenuation, vascular smooth muscle function, and venous pooling in the lower extremities [20,21]. These hemodynamic changes could predispose to atherosclerosis and thrombosis of the lower extremities. Future investigations are needed to allow investigators to develop therapeutic strategies that will prevent the sitting-induced vascular dysfunction. This will be especially beneficial in populations that are more susceptible to prolonged sitting and thus prevent its adverse metabolic and CV effects.

Discussion

The industrial revolution and technological advances have attracted a large number of people from the country and their farming activities to large urbanized cities and have limited their mobility. Today, people spend more than 60% of their 16-hour waking time sitting before computers at work or home, watching TV, speaking on the phone, and commuting from long distance to work sitting for long time in a car in congested highways. Children do not walk to a neighborhood school anymore but are transported by bus or car to distant schools. After school, instead of playing with their friends outside their homes, they spend enormous amount of time playing video games or talking on the phone. Adults do not go to the stores to shop for things they need, but instead order them through the internet to be delivered in their front door. Therefore, it is not surprising that the *Homo Erectus* has now become *Homo Sedentarius* [22]. Before the industrial revolution, 90% of people were agriculturalists, now more than half of the world's population lives in cities and the number is continuously increasing. In addition, urbanization is associated with seated work and the use of automated work and screen-based leisure time and play. Technological changes in people's homes and work places, together with societal trends that contribute to the progression of human inactivity, continue to appear worldwide and it is naïve to assume that we have reached the pinnacle of physical inactivity [23]. Data from a previous NHANES report show that only 28% of Americans are physically active by meeting the minimal exercise recommendations of 30 min/d five times/wk [2,24]. Also, employed persons in many Western countries spend up to a half a day being sedentary and it is time to stem this unhealthy trend [25]. For this reason, the American College of Sports Medicine (ACSM) has issued a recent statement for the professional care providers to recommend daily exercises for their patients [26]. According to this statement, adults should engage in moderate-intensity cardiorespiratory exercise for ≥ 30 min/d for ≥ 5 d/wk for a total of ≥ 150 min/wk or vigorous exercise for ≥ 20 min/d for ≥ 3 d/wk for a total of ≥ 75 min/wk. In addition to exercising regularly, the ACSM recommends to reduce the total time spent in sedentary pursuits. Two recent cross-sectional studies have also demonstrated an association between the number of breaks and various cardiometabolic parameters after accounting for moderate to vigorous PA [27.28]. Sedentary behavior is responsible for CVD, which is the most prevalent modifiable noncommunicable disease worldwide [29]. According to World Health Organization (WHO), CVD accounted in 2019 for 32% of CVD deaths or for 18.2 million deaths worldwide [30]. In order to stem the increase in sedentary behavior, the WHO has issued in 2020 new specific exercise guidelines for children, adolescents, adults, and older adults [31]. According to these guidelines, all adults (16-64 years old) should exercise for 150-300 min/wk with moderate PA or 75-150 min/wk with vigorous PA. Children (5-17 years old, should perform a moderate to vigorous aerobic PA for 60 min/d. Regarding older adults (≥ 65 years of age), the same guidelines for adults are recommended, since all studies on exercise have included all adults. In addition all age groups should perform regularly muscle strengthening exercises. Regarding reduction of sedentary behavior, its reduction is strongly recommended, although the evidence is insufficient to quantify the quantity of sedentary behavior threshold. It is hoped that with the development of wearable monitoring devices, like smart watches, the people will be more aware of their daily activity sedentary time and will try to improve their sedentary behaviors [32].

Conclusion: there is plenty of experimental clinical evidence from controlled clinical as well as prospective cohort studies that prolonged sitting time is associated with several adverse health effects. These include obesity, T2DM, hypertension, CVD, CHD, and death. Unfortunately, sedentary behavior is increasing continuously across all age groups due mostly to increasing urbanization of the population and the advanced technology. Work now can be done at home through the computers instead of going to the office and increases the sitting the daily sitting time. In addition, people spent most of their leisure time at home playing with computers or video games, watching TV and ordering their food or other items through the internet, which are delivered to their doors instead of going to the stores to shop. The children now do not walk to neighbor schools, but are bushed to distant schools. Increased effort should be exercised by the health agencies and doctors to recommend physical activity and decrease the sitting time emphasizing the serious adverse health effects of sedentary behavior. Hopefully, the new wearable devices like smart watches which continuously monitor a person's condition, will stimulate people to modify their daily behaviors and decrease the sitting time.

References

1. Chrysant SG, Chrysant GS. The cardiovascular consequences of excessive sitting time. J Clin Hypertens 2015; 17 528-
2. Matthews CE, Chen KY, Freedson PS, et al. Amount of time spent in sedentary behaviors in the United States 2003-2004. Am J Epidemiol 2008;167: 875- 881

3. Patel AV, Bernstein L, Deka A, et al. Leisure time spent sitting in relation to total mortality in a prospective cohort of US adults. Am J Epidemiol 2010; 172: 419-429
4. Warren TY, Barry V, Hooker SP, et al. Sedentary behaviors increase risk of cardiovascular disease mortality in men. Med Sci Sports Exerc 2010; 121: 879-885
5. Dunstan DW, Barr EL, Healy GN, et al. Television viewing time and mortality. The Australian Diabetes Obesity and Lifestyle Study. (AusDiab). Circulation 2010; 121: 384- 391
6. Wijndaele K, Brage S, Besson H, et al. Television viewing and incident cardiovascular disease: prospective associations and mediation analysis in the EPIC Norfolk Study. PloS One 2011; 6: e20058
7. Stamatakis E, Hamer M, Dunstan DW. Screen-based entertainment time, all-cause mortality, and cardiovascular events. J AM Coll Cardiol 2011; 57: 292- 299
8. Ford FS. Combined television viewing and computer use and mortality from all-causes and diseases of the circulatory system among adults in the United States. BMC Public Health 2012; 12: 70
9. Matthews CE, George SM, Moore SC, et al. Amount of time spent in specific behaviors and cause-specific mortality in US adults. Am J Clin Nutr 2012; 95: 437- 445
10. Ford ES, Caspersen CJ. Sedentary behavior and cardiovascular disease: a review of prospective studies. Int J Epidemiol 2012; 41: 1338- 1353

11. Dunstan DW, Howard B, Healy GN. Too much sitting: a health hazard. Diabetes Res Clin Pract 2012; 97: 368- 376
12. Shuval K, Finley CE, Barlow CE, et al. Sedentary behavior, cardiorespiratory fitness, physical activity, and cardiometabolic risk in men: the Cooper Center Longitudinal Study. Mayo Clin Proc 2014; 89: 1052- 1062
13. Kulinski JP, Khera A, Ayers CR, et al. association between cardiorespiratory fitness and accelerometer-derived physical activity and sedentary time in the general population. Mayo Clin Proc 2014; 89: 106 – 1071
14. Pandey A, Sahuddin U, Garg S, et al. Continuous dose-response association between sedentary time and risk for cardiovascular disease. A meta-analysis. JAMA Cardiol 2016; 1: 575- 583
15. Lansitie M, Kangas M, Jokelainen J, et al. Cardiovascular disease risk and all-cause mortality associated with accelerometer-measured physical activity and sedentary time-a prospective population-based study in older adults. BMC Geriatrics 2022; 22: 729
16. Zderic TW, Hamilton MT. Physical inactivity amplifies the sensitivity of skeletal muscle in lipid-induced downregulation of lipoprotein lipase activity. J Appl Physiol 2006; 100: 249- 257
17. Hamilton MT, Hamilton DG, Zderic TW. Role of low energy expenditure and sitting in obesity, metabolic syndrome, type 2 diabetes, and cardiovascular diseases. Diabetes 2007; 56:2655- 2667

18. Pekas EJ, Allen MF, Park SY. Prolonged sitting and peripheral vascular function: potential mechanisms and methodological considerations. J Appl Physiol 2023; 134: 810- 822
19. Chao Y, Ye P, Zhu L, et al. Low shear stress induces endothelial reactive oxygen species via ATIR/eNOS/NO pathway. J Cell Physiol 2018; 233: 1384-1395
20. Taylor FC, Pinto AJ, Maniar N, et al. The acute effects of prolonged uninterrupted sitting on vascular function: a systematic review and meta-analysis. Med Sci Sports Exerc 2022; 54: 67- 76
21. Liu H, O'Brien MW, Wu Y, et al. An acute bout of prolonged sitting blunts popliteal endothelium-independent dilation in young, healthy adults. J Appl Physiol 2023; 134: 521- 528
22. Levine JA. Lethal sitting: homo sedentarius seeks answers. Physiology 2014; 29: 300- 301
23. Boakye K, Bovbjerg M, Schuna J, Jr, et al. Urbanization and physical activity in the global perspective urban and rural epidemiology study. Scientific Rep 2023; 13: 290
24. Kruger J, Yore MM, Kohl HW 3rd. Leisure-time physical activity patterns by weight control status 1999-2002 NHANES. Med Sci Sports Exerc 2007; 39: 788- 795
25. Van Uffern JG, Wong J, Chau JY, et al. Occupational sitting and health risks: a systematic review. Am J Prev Med 2010; 39: 379- 388
26. Garber CE, Blissmer B, Deschenes MR, et al. Quantity and quality of exercise for developing and maintaining cardiorespiratory, musculoskeletal, and neuromotor

fitness in apparently healthy adults: guidelines for prescribing exercise. Med Sci Sports Exerc 2011; 43: 1334- 1359

27. Healy GN, Dunstan DW, Salmon J, et al. Breaks in sedentary time: beneficial associations with metabolic risk. Diabetes Care 2008; 31: 661- 666
28. Healy GN, Matthews CE, Dunstan DW, et al. Sedentary time and cardiometabolic risk. Eur Heart J 2011; 32: 590- 597
29. Yang Z, Chen S, Bao R, et al. Public health concern on sedentary behavior and cardiovascular disease: a bibliometric analysis of literature from 1990 to 2022. Medicina 2022; 58: 1764
30. Roth GA, Mensah GA, Johnson CO, et al. Global burden of cardiovascular diseases and risk factors, 1990-2019: update from the GBD 2019 study. J Am Coll Cardiol 2020; 76: 2982- 3021
31. Bull FC, Al-Ansari SS, Biddle S, et al. World Health Organization 2020 guidelines on physical activity and sedentary behaviour. Br J Sports Med 2020; 54: 1451-1462
32. Kang HS, Exworthy M. Wearing the future-wearables to empower users to take greater responsibility for their health and care: a scoping review. JMIR Mhealth Uhealth 2022; 10: e35664

Table 1

Adverse Cardiovascular Consequences of Prolonged Sitting Time

Author	Study (type)	Subjects (no)	Age (yrs)	F-U (yrs)	CV Events (kind)	Statistical (significance)

Patel [3]	Prosp	113,216	63-65	14	CVM RR 1,17M,1.34W
Warren [4]	Prosp	7744	20-89	21	CVM $p < 0.001$
Dunstan [5]	Prosp	8800	49-57	6.6	CVM HR 1.80, 1.46 ACM
Wijndaele [6]	Prosp	12,608	61.4	6.9	CVM HR 1.06
Stamatakis [7]	Prosp	4512	57-60	4.3	ACM HR 2.30
Ford [8]	Prosp	7350	44-67	5.8	CVD, HR 1.17
Matthews [9]	Prosp	240,818	50-71	na	ACM, CVM HR 1.47, 2.00
Shuval [12]	Prosp	1269	46.2	8.5	TG/HDL ratio $p < 0.05$
Kulinski [13]	Prosp	2223	22.4	na	PF $p = 0.03$M, < 0.001W
Pandey [14]	Rev-Meta	720,125	54.5	11	CVD $p < 0.001$
Lansitie [15]	Prosp	660	68.9	6.2	FRS $\beta - 0.779$, $p < 0.001$

F-U = follow-up, prosp = prospective study, Rev-Meta = review and meta-analysis, CVM = cardiovascular mortality, ACM = all-cause mortality, TG/HDL ratio = triglyceride/HDL ratio, PF = physical fitness, FRS = Framingham risk score. The statistics are for the greatest sitting time.

Chapter Two

Beneficial Cardiovascular Effects of Physical Activity and Trajectories of Physical Activity

Introduction

As reported previously, prolonged physical inactivity is unhealthy and associated with adverse CV effects [1-11]. In contrast, regular PA of grades and forms is associated with improvement in CV health and reduction of the incidence several CV complications demonstrated by many studies [12-26]. In addition, PA is beneficial in older and frail people [27-30]. In order to get a current information on the different types of PA and trajectories of PA and their effects on CV health, CVD and mortality, a Medline search of the English literature was conducted between 2015 and 2022 and 60 pertinent papers were selected. The information from these papers in combination with collateral literature will be discussed.

Cardiovascular Benefits of Physical Activity

The great majority of studies have shown a beneficial and protective effect of PA on CVD, CHD and death [12-26]. The data from these studies are summarized in table 1 and they will, briefly, discussed here. The study Lear et al [12], evaluated the different types and duration of PA on the incidence of CVD and mortality in a large prospective multinational study involving 130,843 subjects mean age 50.2 ± 9.7 years, free of CVD at baseline. They found a positive association an association with reduction of in the incidence of mortality with the different levels of PA. After a mean follow-up of 6.9 years, the highest level of PA was associated with significant reduction in mortality, HR o,80 (95% CI 0.74-0.87, $p < 0.0001$) and CVD, HR 0.86 (95% CI 0.78-0.93, $p < 0.001$). Also, higher physical activity was associated with lower incidence of CVD and mortality in higher, middle, and low income countries. The study by Moholdt et al [13], was a similar prospective study of 3307 participants on the effects of levels of PA on all-cause mortality and CVD risk and weight loss in patients with CHD. After a mean follow-up of 30 years, there was a lower risk for all-cause mortality in patients maintaining a low of high PA, adjusted HR, 0.81 (95% CI 0.67-0.97) and 0.64 (95% CI 0.50-0.83), respectively. With respect to weight changes, weight loss ≥ o.10 kg/m^{2}/year was associated with significant increase in all-cause mortality, aHR 1.30 (95% CI 1.12-1.50), but not weight gain ≥ 0.10 kg/m$^{2/}$/year. In another study, Xu and Cao [14], analyzed the results of a prospective study of 356,967 participants from the UK Biobank, ages 37-73 years on the effects of PA on mortality in subjects with several cardiometabolic risk factors at baseline. After a mean follow-up of 13 years, subjects exercising ≥ 2 times/wk had a multivariable HR 2.57 (95% CI 2.38-2.78) risk for mortality compared with those normal cardiometabolic risk profile, HR 1.58 (95% CI 1.50-1.66). In another prospective study Kim et al [15], analyzed the effects of different types of PA on mortality in 58,537 participants from the Korean National insurance service mean age 73.9 ± 5,8 years. After a follow-up of 3.3 years, the incidence of all-cause mortality was decreased by 26%, HR 0.74 (95% CI 0.68-0.82) in those with light PA, by 27%, HR 0.73 (95% CI 0.63-0.84) in those with light to moderate PA, and by 34%, HR 0.66 (95% CI 0,54-0.79) in those with moderate PA compared to those with sedentary existence. The study by Corczyga et al [16], is a prospective study of different levels of PA on the incidence of all-cause mortality in 1389 postmenopausal women ages 50-79 years with a previous MI. After 3-6 years of follow-up, increased PA was associated with a decrease in all-cause mortality, HR 0.54 (95% CI 0.34-0.86) and HR 0.52 (95% CI 0.36-0.73) for those maintaining high PA. In contrast, prolonged sitting was associated with a 9% increase in all-cause mortality, HR 1.09 (95% CI 1.01-1.19). In a similar study Eckblom et al [17], examined the effects of different types of PA on all-cause mortality in 22,227 Swedish patients ages 60.8-62.0 years with a previous MI. After a mean follow-up of 4.2 years, and adjustment for important confounders, the mortality was greatly reduced in those being constantly active, HR 0.29 (95% CI 0.21-0.41), and 0.41 (95% CI 0.31-0.55) for those with increased PA, and 0.56 (95% CI0.45-0.69) for those remaining constantly inactive. In their study Wanamethee eta l [18], investigated the different types and levels of PA on all-cause mortality in 5934 older men mean age 63 years with established CHD. After 5 years of follow-up, the assigned scores of PA were 1 for inactive to ≥ 21 for vigorous PA. The fully adjusted RR for all-cause mortality and CV mortality were, 0.42 (95% CI 0.25-0.71) for light PA, 0.47 (95% CI 0.24-0.92) for moderate PA, and 0.63 (95% CI 0.39-1.03) for vigorous PA compared to inactivity. Mes who started light PA later in the study, also had lower incidence of all-cause mortality, RR 0.58 (95% CI 0.33-1.03) than those who stayed inactive. In this study, non-sporting PA was more beneficial than sporting activity. In another similar study, Steffen-Batey, et al {19] examined the effects of different levels of

PA on the risk of mortality and reinfarction in 406 Mexican and non-Hispanic men and women ages 58.4-64.1 years. After 7 years of follow-up, the RR of mortality was 0.21 (95% CI 0.10-0.44) for the active non-change group, 0.11 (95% CI 0.03-0.40) for the increased activity group, and 0.49 (95% CI 0.26-0.90) for the decreased activity group. The RRs for reinfarction were 0.40 (95% CI 0.24-0.66) for the active group, 0,22 (95% CI 0.09-0.50) for the increased activity group, and 0.93 (95% CI 0.59-1.43) for the sedentary group. The study by Buckley et al [20], is a retrospective study of 18,383 patients mean age 64.8 years with a chronic coronary syndrome (CCS). This study evaluated the effects of cardiac rehabilitation (CR) compared to percutaneous coronary intervention (PCI) on all-cause mortality, rehospitalization, and CV morbidities (acute MI, stroke, or new onset HF). After 1.5 years of follow-up, the odds ratio (OR) of CR vs PCI was 0.37(95% CI 0.29-0.47) for all-cause mortality, 0.29 (95% CI 0.27-0.32) for rehospitalization, and CV morbidities. The patients that receive CR + PCI, the OR was not significantly different for all-cause mortality, OR 1.00 (95% CI 0.63-1.60), rehospitalization, OR 1.00 (95% CI 0.82-1.32, AMI, OR 1.11 (95% CI 0.68-1.81), and stroke, OR 0.71 (95% CI 0.39-1.31) compared to CR only. In a population-based study, Kang et al [21] analyzed the effects of different types and levels of PA on all-cause mortality and non-CV mortality in 6076 Korean subjects mean age 72.0 years. After a median follow-up of 3.8 years, the weighted all-cause mortality rate was 4.8, 4.6, 3.5, and 2.9/100 person years in persistent non-exercisers, exercise dropouts, new exercisers, and exercise maintainers, respectively. The all-cause mortality was lower in new exercisers, HR 0.73 (95%

CI 0.58-0.91) and in exercise maintainers, HR 0,53 (95% CI 0.38-0.71). Exercise maintainers had also, lower risk for CV mortality, HR 0.34 (95% CI 0.17-0.64). Also, the risk of CV mortality was lower in new exercisers compared to persistent non-exercisers ($p < 0.001$).

Cardiovascular effects of exercise trajectories

The study by Mok et al [22], is a prospective population-based study evaluated the effects of physical activity energy expenditure (PAEE) trajectories on CVD and all-cause mortality 14,599 subjects ages 40-79 years. The self-reported PA was categorized as none, 0.1-3.5, 3,6-7.0, and ≥ 7.0 hours/week. After a median follow-up of 12.5 years, for each 1 kj/kg/d/year increase in PAEE (equivalent to a trajectory of being inactive at baseline and gradually increase the PAEE over 5 years, meeting the WHO requirements of 150 mi/week), was associated with a decrease in all-cause mortality and CV mortality, HR 0.76 (95% CI 0.71-0.82) and 0.71 (95% CI 0.62-0.82) adjusted for CV risk factors, respectively. Also, a joint analysis of baseline physical PA and trajectories of PA compared to physically inactive subjects, showed that those with increasing PA trajectories over time experienced a lower risk of all-cause mortality, HR 0.58 (95% CI 0.43-0.78). This study showed that middle age adults with or without CVD can gain substantial longevity by being more physically active. In another prospective study, Aggio et al [23] investigated the different types and levels of PA trajectories on all-cause mortality in 3231 men ages 40-59 years of age. After a mean follow-up of 16.4 years, subjects with high/stable PA and moderate/increased PA, had lower all-cause mortality, HR 0.83 (95% CI 0.74-

0.94) and 0.76 (95% CI 0.66-0.88), respectively compared with hose with low/decreased PA. In addition, a dose-response association with CV benefits was noted in middle to older age subjects. Also, In a prospective study Marques Elias et al [24], evaluated the PA trajectories on CV risk in 417 subjects mean age 48.4 years. After 4 years of follow-up, the trajectories of moderate/stable and high/stable PA were associated with lower CV risk than those with normal/stable trajectories ($p < 0.05$). The subjects that benefited from the PA trajectories had also LDL-C and obesity levels. Similarly, Berbiellini Amidei et al [25], investigated the different types and levels of PA trajectories on the risk of CVD in 3099 older subjects mean age 74.4 years, of whom 1037 had preexisting CVD. After 7 years of follow-up, men with stable/high PA had a significantly lower risk for CV outcomes than those with stable/low PA, HR o.48 (95% CI 0.27-0.86, $p_{for\ trend} = 0.002$). In addition, the HRs after adjustments for CV risk factors were, o74 (95% CI 0.58-0.94) for CVD, 0.66 (95% CI 0.50-0.87) for CHD, 0.72 (95% CI 0.53-0.98) for HF, and 1.02 (95% CI 0.69-1.52) for stroke. Also, in a systematic review Gonzales-Jaramillo et al [26], assessed the effects of different exercise trajectories on all-cause mortality in 33,576 patients with CHD mean age 62.5 years. The PA status was categorized as inactive, active, increased, and decreased over time. After a maximum follow-up of 15.7 years, the all-cause mortality was 50%, 45%, and 20% lower in those who stayed active, HR0.50 (95% CI 0.39-0.63), 0.55 (95% CI 0.44-0.70), and 0.80 (95% CI 0.64-0.99), respectively. Similar results were observed for CV mortality, except those who decreased their PA, HR 0.91 (95 CI 0.67-1.24). The results from these studies are also summarized in table 1.

Factors Mediating the Beneficial Cardiovascular effects of Exercise

Clinical and experimental studies have demonstrated that the beneficial CV effects of exercise are mediated through favorable modifications of several metabolic as well as clinical CV risk factors. These factors are depicted in fig. 1

Metabolic Factors

Insulin and Glucose Homeostasis: Several studies have shown the beneficial CV effects of PA being meditated through increase in insulin sensitivity [31-34]. Vigorous PA increases insulin sensitivity such as in endurance athletes, which is almost eliminated within 38-48 hours of exercise cessation [31]. Also, regular PA is associated with increase insulin resistance and a decrease in the MetS syndrome and T2DM [32]. These effects are mediated through muscle contraction, increase in AMPK and GLUTA4 resulting in increased glucose uptake by the exercising muscle. Endurance athletes studied after cessation of PA for 60 min, 12 hours and 7 days, showed a glucose clearance by the euglycemic clamp of 15.6 ± 2 ml/kg/min 12 hours after the last bout of PA compared to 7.8 ml/kg/min of a sedentary control group. After refraining from PA for 60 hr and 7 days, the glucose clearance decreased to 10.1 ± 1.0 ml/kg/min and 8.5 ± 0.5 ml/kg/min, respectively [32]. Also, activities such as walking, cycling, jogging, swimming, rely primarily on energy provided by glucose utilization mediated through increase in insulin sensitivity [33]. Other studies have shown that the skeletal muscle accounts for 40% of the total body mass, and plays a critical role in metabolic homeostasis. Under increased PA could dispose up to 80% of glucose under insulin simulated conditions [34]. This effect is mediated through GLUTA4 across the cell membranes and intracellular glucose metabolism and are reversed quickly after cessation of exercise [35]. With an increased and prolonged exercise, the skeletal muscle shifts its energy requirements from glucose to fatty acids [36]. This is mediated through GLUTA4 across cell membranes and intracellular glucose metabolism. Recent advances in proteomics have uncovered several signaling pathways involved in muscle glucose uptake, such as activated protein kinase (AMPK), protein kinase activity (PKA), calmodulin mediated kinase (CaMK) and mitogen activated protein kinase (MAPK), among others [36]. Another study found a more complex signaling pathway in glucose utilization and homeostasis mediated through a complex signaling pathway involving the kinases AMPK, PKA, CaMK, MAPK, PKC, FAK, and mTOR [37].

Lipid Metabolism: The beneficial cardiovascular effects of exercise can also, be mediated through its favorable actions on lipid metabolism by decreasing total cholesterol, LDL-C, VLDL-C, triglycerides, and increasing the HDL-C levels and particle size [38,39]. Habitual exercise also reduces the levels of cholesterol transport protein (CETP) and increases the muscle lipoprotein lipase (LPL) content and activity and increase the hydrolysis of triglycerides [40,41]. Recent studies have also shown that exercise-induced increase in HDL-C is associated with an elevation of liver X receptors (LXRs) leading to the expression of genes involved in the regulation of cholesterol homeostasis [42]. In addition to changes in plasma lipids, exercise can directly impact the arterial wall homeostasis and prevent the progression of atherosclerosis and reduce the incidence of CHD as has been demonstrated in active compared to sedentary individuals [42].

Branched-Chain Aminoacids: Emerging evidence suggests that branched-chain aminoacids (BCAA) are involved in the pathogenesis of CVD, myocardial infarction (MI), ischemia-reperfusion injury, and HF and are a hallmark of metabolic disorders, including obesity, insulin resistance and T2DM [43-46]. They exert their effects through activation of serine/threonine protein kinase mTOR, mitochondrial dysfunction, shifts in cardiac substrate utilization, and platelet activation [47].

Exerkines: Recent clinical and experimental evidence suggests that the beneficial CV effects of exercise could be mediated through an increase in the release of exerkines. Exerkines are defined as signaling moieties that are released in response to acute and chronic exercise and mediate their effects through endocrine, paracrine, or autocrine pathways [48]. They are released from multiple organs in the body including skeletal muscles (myokines), heart muscles (cardiokines), liver (hepatokines), white adipose tissue (adipokines), brown adipose tissue (batokines), and neurons (neurokines). Their potential roles, involve treatment of CVD, T2DM, obesity, and healthy ageing [49]. At present, the contribution of exercise to CV protection is under intense investigation by NHLBI to discover the molecular transducers that underlie the effects of exercise on exerkines release [50]. During exercise, there is a crosstalk among many organs and cells mediated by many biomolecules secreted in response to exercise. In this regard, the role of skeletal muscle has been shown to be the largest secretory organ of specific myokines [51]. The classic exerkines released during acute exercise, include IL-6, and IL-8 [52]. Il-6-6 serves as a metabolic coordinator during acute exercise by regulating lipolysis in adipose tissue and hepatic glucose production and utilization by the skeletal muscle. It may also be involved in cardiac remodeling in endurance training linked to left ventricular hypertrophy in these situations [53]. IL-8 is primarily known for its angiogenic activity, endothelial cell proliferation and capillary extension through the CXC receptor 2 expressed in endothelial cells [54].

Endothelial Function: Regular exercise has been shown to attenuate arterial stiffness and improve endothelial function. Its effects are mediated through changes in endothelial regulation of vascular smooth muscle tone and structural changes in vascular media by decreasing collagen deposition and increasing the vascular elastic content [55]. The decrease in vascular stiffness with exercise results in a decrease in central aortic systolic blood pressure and pulse pressure and decreases their detrimental CV effects, especially in older subjects [56-58]. In addition, exercise results in an increased release of nitric oxide (NO), which exerts vasorelaxant and vasodilatory effects resulting in increased myocardial blood flow and reduction of CVD and mortality [59]. Additional beneficial CV effects of exercise are mediated through mitochondrial adaptations from the vascular stress stimulating NO synthase activity increasing NO production with increase in vascular plasticity and ameliorating vascular dysfunction of advancing age. Also, the mitochondrial adaptations to exercise improve the bioenergetics, the balance of redox status, and ameliorate the vascular dysfunction of improve vascular health [60].

Autophagy: Autophagy or (self eating in Greek), is an evolutionary intracellular catalytic process that eliminates degraded cellular structures including mitochondria and plays a significant in body homeostasis and its activity is increased with exercise [61-65]. In addition, several studies have shown that the exercise mediated beneficial CV effects could be mediated through an increase in the activity of autophagy [66-68]. Autophagy exerts its beneficial CV effects through transportation of intracellular damaged and denatured proteins and mitochondria into liposomes for degradation and digestion and thus improves the function of healthy myocardial cells [69]. There are three major types of autophagy, macroautophagy, microaurtophagy and chaperon mediated autophagy (CMA). Macroautophagy exerts its effects through the formation of double-membrane vesicles called autophagosome and engulfs damaged, dysfunctional and redundant proteins and organelles. The sequestered cargo is then delivered to liposomes for degradation. Microphagy involves a direct engulfment of cytoplasmic cargo including mitochondria for degradation by liposomes. The CMA entails the recognition of soluble proteins translocated across the liposomal membrane for degradation with the assistance of the CMA receptor. Generally, autophagy contributes to the maintenance of cellular function and survival in all living organisms and involves multiple signaling pathways [70]. Among them, the most well studied are the Class I Phosphoinositide 3 kinase and the rapamycin (mTOR) signaling pathways. With respect to CV protection, experimental research evidence links autophagy to prevention of CV disorders [71]. In temporary or permanent occlusion of a coronary artery the lack of oxygen and nutrient supply to cardiomyocytes imposes lethal consequences and in this setting efficient autophagic response allows the cardiomyocytes to cope with ischemic and nutritional stress. On the other hand, alterations in the function of autophagy and mitophagy have been associated with several cardiomyopathies [70].

Clinical Factors

Besides the metabolic factors there are several clinical factors that contribute to the beneficial effects of exercise.

Obesity: Obesity is major health problem and is rising globally with an estimated incidence of 573 to safer from obesity and T2DM by the year 2030 [71-73]. In addition, obesity is associated with several CV risk factors such as metabolic syndrome, hypertension, and dyslipidemia. In this regard, regular PA has been associated with a decreased incidence of T2DM, hypertension, dyslipidemia and CVD [74-76]. Overweight and obesity are defined with a body mass index (BMI) of 25-29.9 kg/m^3 and BMI ≥ 30 kg/m^3, respectively [77]. Maintenance of normal body weight is associated with reduced incidence of CV complications and death in both men and women [78-84]. In the pathological determinants of atherosclerosis in the youth study, atherosclerotic lesions were observed only in those subjects with thick abdominal panniculus, indicating the fundamental role of central obesity in the development of atherosclerotic disease [85].

Metabolic Syndrome: The metabolic syndrome (MetS) is defined by the National Cholesterol Education Program (NCEP) as a cluster of 3 or more of 5 risk CV factors. These factors include central obesity (waist circumference > 102 cm in men, 88 cm in women), elevated triglycerides (≥ 150 mg/dl), low HDL-C (< 40 mg/dl) in men, (< 50 mg/dl) in women, increased fasting glucose levels (≥ 110 mg/dl), and increased BP (≥ 130/85 mmHg). Due to these risk factors, the MetS is associated with an increased incidence of T2DM, CVD, CHD, and death [86-91]. Obesity and MetS frequently overlap in the literature and is designated as unhealthy obesity, since 35-50% of obese subjects do not have the MetS [92,93].

Diabetes Mellitus. T2DM is also a major risk factor for CVD, CHD, hypertension, and mortality due mostly to its macrovascular and microvascular adverse effects [95-96], and its incidence is growing fast worldwide. It is expected that its incidence is projected to increase from the current 537 million of persons 20-79 years of age to grow to 643 million in 2030 and to 783 million in 2045 [97]. Therefore, prevention and treatment of T2DM is critical to reduce its CV adverse effects. Among the means to achieve this, are lifestyle changes with exercise and healthy diet in addition to pharmacotherapy if necessary [98-100], which decrease the glucose levels and prevent the postprandial hyperglycemia and its detrimental CV effects. Recent studies have shown the beneficial effects of exercise on the incidence of T2DM and the mechanism of action mediated through in mitochondrial dysfunction and autophagy [101-103]. The mitochondrion lies at the intersection of critical cellular pathways involving energy substrate metabolism, generation of reactive oxygen species (ROS), and apoptosis resulting in downstream deficits in organ function involving the myocardium and other organs. Regular aerobic exercise increases insulin sensitivity and improves muscular mitochondrial function [102]. In addition, exercise by reducing the hyperglycemia decreases the oxidative stress and improves the reparative process of autophagy, increases β-cell function, insulin production, and improves myocardial contraction [103]. Also, reduction of HbA_{1c} of < 7% prevents the rise in oxidative stress and improves the altered mitochondrial morphology and autophagy [103]. As has been stated previously, autophagy is an intracellular catabolic process that leads to sequestration of cellular debris and damaged organelles and improves CV health. Thus, exercise prevents and corrects the mitochondrial abnormalities and improves the diabetic status [104].

Hypertension: Hypertension is considered a major risk factor for CVD, CHD, HF, stroke, and death. Several large reviews and meta-analyses have demonstrated that hypertension is associated with an increase in CVD and mortality and reduction of high BP prevents or decreases the adverse CV effects of high BP [105-109]. In a systematic review and meta-analysis by Etehad et al [105] of 123 studies involving 613,815 participants, a meta-regression analysis showed that for every 10 mmHg reduction of BP was associated with a decrease in CVD, RR 0.80 (95% CI 0.77-0.83), CHD, RR 0.83 (95% CI 0.78-0.88), stroke, RR 0.73 (95% CI 0.68-0.77), and HF, RR 0.72 (95% CI 0.67-0.78), and all-cause mortality, RR 0.87 (95% CI 0.84-0.91). In another review and meta-analysis by Brunston and Calberg [106] of 74 trials representing 306,273 subjects, reduction of SBP was associated with reduced risk of major CV events, RR 0.78 (95% CI 0.70-0.87) and risk of death, RR 0.93 (95% CI 0.87-1.00). Similarly, in another major review and meta-analysis by Luo et al [107] of 17 observational cohorts involving 4.5 million young adults with an average follow-up of 14.7 years, a graded progressive association was found between the BP categories and increased risk of CV events. High normal BP was associated with an increased CV risk, RR 1.35 (95% CI 1.22-1.49), grade 1 hypertension RR 1.92 (95% CI 1.68-2.19), and grade 2 hypertension, RR 3.15 (95% CI 2.31-4.29). Similar results were observed for CHD and stroke. However, the number needed to treat to prevent for 1 year to prevent one CV events was 2672 for participants with normal BP, 1450 for those with high normal BP, 552 for those with grade 1 hypertension, and 236 for those with grade 2 hypertension. Also, in major data analysis by the Blood Pressure Lowering Treatment Trialists Collaboration of 48 randomized trials involving 344,716 participants [108], reduction of SBP was associated with a decrease incidence of major CV events was 31.9 (95% CI 31.3- 32.5) per 1000/person years. In participants with preexisting CVD, major CVD events occurred in 39.7 (95% CI 39.0-40.5) per 1000/person years, compared to the comparator group of 36.0 (95% CI 35.3-36.7). In another study, Flint et al [109] analyzed the data from 1.3 million adults from the general population. They found that after an 8 year follow-up, SBP > - 140 mmHg was associated with increased incidence of adverse CV outcomes (MI, ischemic or hemorrhagic stroke), HR 1.18 (95% CI 1.17-1.80) and for DBP >- 90 mmHg, HR 1.06 (95% CI 1.06-1.07). In this study the SBP was more important than the DBP in the incidence of adverse CV events. Thus, reduction of BP is very critical for the prevention of hypertension mediated adverse CV events. In this regard exercise has been very effective in reducing the BP either alone or in combination with pharmacologic therapy [110-114]. Several studies have demonstrated the independent BP reducing effects of exercise. In a review and meta-analysis by Fu et al [110] of 14 studies involving 1027 patients, showed that aerobic training resulted in significant reduction of SBP and DBP, waited mean difference (WMD) of - 9'91 mmHg (95% CI – 14.21 to – 5.61, p < 0.0001) compared to the control group and WMD – 4.32 (95% CI - 7.02 to – 1.62, p < 0.0001) compared to control group for the SBP and DBP, respectively. In another review and meta-analysis, Saco-Ledo et al [111] examined the effects of exercise in 10 studies involving 380 participants with resistant hypertension. Analysis of results showed that an acute bout of exercise temporarily reduced the BP, where as more prolonged exercise (8-12 weeks) reduced significantly the 24 hr ABP – 9.9 mmHg (95% CI – 15.4 to – 4.4) for SBP and – 5.0 mmHg (95% CI – 7.0 to – 3.0) for the DBP. The daytime ABP was reduced by -11.7 mmHg (95% CI – 17..8 to – 5.7) for

SBP and – 7.4 mmHg (95% CI -11.9 to – 2.0) for DBP. Another review and meta-analysis by Wen and Wang [112], of 13 studies involving 802 hypertensive patients. Aerobic exercise resulted in significant reductions in SBP and DBP compared t o the control group. In single center study Arciero et al [113], studied the effects of time of exercise in 27 women and 20 men on BP and abdominal fat reduction. The study showed that AM exercise reduced the abdominal and BP, where as evening exercise improved the muscular performance in women. In contrast, in men PM exercise reduced the SBP and fatigue. In another single center study, Dimeo et al [114] investigated the effects of exercise on BP in 50 patients with resistant to treatment hypertension. Exercise reduced the SBP and DBP by 24 hr ABPM by 6 ± 12 mmHg and by 3 ± 7 mmHg respectively.

Cardiovascular Remodeling: Among the many CV benefits of exercise are its beneficial effects on cardiovascular remodeling. This effect is mediated through changes in cardiac structure, cardiac mass, cardiac geometry, and function in both young and old hearts [115]. Morphologically, the sedentary aged heart undergoes several morphological and functional changes, such as LVH, increased myocyte cell, size, and decreased ventricular size [116- 118]. Autopsies of the human heart show higher deposits of collagen in subjects older than 65 years compared to younger subjects 20-35 years of age, even without underlying cardiac disease [119]. Similar changes in cardiac morphology have also been shown in experimental animals [120]. These structural changes of the heart are associated with diastolic dysfunction with impaired relaxation and diminished ability to respond to cardiac work due to diminished inotropic and chronotropic reserve [118]. The exercise-induced increase in cardiac size in athletes with enlarged atrial and left ventricular dimensions are of the so called physiologic type and are not associated with myocardial dysfunction [121]. Clinical evidence also, suggests that exercise-induced cardiac hypertrophy increases the systolic function of the heart in previously sedentary subjects and improves their aerobic exercise performance [122,123]. The long-term benefits of exercise have been attributed to its multiple clinical and molecular cardiac adaptations associated with improvement in the quality of life and prolongation of the life span [124,125].

Comment

The health benefits of exercise on health and disease have been known since antiquity, with Hippokates (460-370 BC) being the first physician to issue written instructions about exercise and its health benefits stating that "eating alone will not keep man well, he must also, take exercise" [126]. In addition, Herodickus, considered the father of sports medicine, recommended to his patients to follow strict diet and regular exercise for good body health [127]. In modern times, regular exercise is a basic requirement for the maintenance of good health and longevity due mostly to its beneficial CV effects as well as its beneficial cardiometabolic effects. In addition, exercise has been used successfully as a diagnostic tool for future incidence of HFrEF and HFpEF in vulnerable patients with T2DM and hypertension [128-132]. Patients with uncomplicated T2DM and hypertension who show an abnormal imaging cardiopulmonary exercise test (CPET) and exercise echocardiography test with reduced peak oxygen uptake (VO_{2peak}) have an increased possibility of developing heart failure in the future and indicate measures to be taken to avoid these complications. Decreased VO_{2peak} indicates underlying myocardiogenic, myogenic, vasculogenic, and neurogenic abnormalities. Also, the importance of exercise in maintaining a healthy lifestyle has been emphasized by recent guidelines from various scientific societies advocating the health benefits of regular exercise [37-39]. Another very important recent finding about exercise is the demonstration by several studies of the exercise trajectories demonstrating a dose-response association of PA and its CV benefits [22-25]. The investigators in these studies analyzed the results with identifiable CVD by comparing the intensity and types of PA over time on the incidence of CV events [22]. Also, the effects of different trajectories and types of PA on CV outcomes (CVD, CHD) compared to the sedentary subjects [22-24]. In addition, a recent study showed the different levels of PA trajectories on all-cause mortality by demonstrating that the over all-cause mortality was decreased by 50%, 45%, and 20% in subjects who remained constantly active, in those who were active and became inactive, and in those who were active and became inactive, compared to constantly sedentary subjects [25]. Further, another study has demonstrated that the time of day that exercise is performed, is not very important, since the CV benefits were similar for hose exercising in the morning versus those exercising in the evening [40]. The mechanism for the cardiovascular benefits of exercise is multifactorial and mediated through metabolic and clinical factors depicted in fig,1. Currently, there is a holistic approach regarding the primary as well as the secondary CV benefits of any type of PA for being fundamental means for CV health and longevity [132]. Therefore, is very critical that physicians should strongly recommend to their patients to constantly physically active and in those that inactive to be active, because the studies have shown even late starters stand to benefit from any type of PA including jogging, walking, bicycling, or gardening.

Figure Legend

Favorable modification of cardiovascular risk factors with exercis

Figure 1. This figure depicts the favorable modification of exercise on several cardiovascular risk factors.

References

1. Chrysant SG, Chrysant GS. The cardiovascular consequences of excess sitting time. J Clin Hypertens 2015; 17: 528- 531
2. Patel AV, Bernstein L, Deka A, et al. Leisure time spent sitting in relation to total mortality in a prospective study of US adults. Am J Epidemiol 2010; 172: 419-429
3. Warren TY, Barry V, Hooker SP, et al. Sedentary behaviors increase risk of cardiovascular disease mortality in men. Med Sci Sports Exerc 2010; 42: 879-885
4. Dustan DW, Barr EL, Healy GN, et al. Television viewing time and mortality. The Australian diabetes, obesity and lifestyle study (AusDiab). Circulation 2010; 121: 384- 391
5. Ford ES. Combined television time and computer use and mortality from all-causes and diseases of the circulatory system among adults in the United States. BMC Public Health 2012; 12: 70
6. Ford ES, Caspersen CJ. Sedentary behavior and cardiovascular disease: a review of prospective studies. Int J Epidemiol 2012; 41: 1338- 1353

7. Shuval K, Finley CE, Barlow CE, et al. Sedentary behavior, cardiorespiratory fitness, physical activity and cardiometabolic risk in men: the Cooper center longitudinal study. Mayo Clin Proc 2014; 89: 1052- 1062
8. Chrysant SG, Chrysant GS. Association of physical activity and trajectories of physical activity with cardiovascular disease. Expert Rev Crdiovasc Ther 2023; 21: 87- 96
9. Chrysant SG, Chrysant GS. Healthy lifestyle could reduce the onset of first heart attack by 80%. J Clin Hypertens 2015; 17: 168-171
10. Lavie CJ, Church TS, Milani RV, et al. Impact of physical activity, cardiorespiratory fitness, and exercise training on markers of inflammation. J Cardiopulm Rehabil Prev 2011; 31: 137- 145
11. Lear SA, Yusuf S. Physical activity to prevent cardiovascular disease. A simple low-cost, and widely applicable approach for all populations. JAM Cardiol 2017; 2: 1358- 1360
12. Lear SA, Hu W, Rangarajan S, et al. The effect of physical activity on mortality and cardiovascular disease in 130,000 people from 17 high-income, middle-income, and low-income countries: the PURE study. Lancet 2017; 390: 2643-2654
13. Moholdt T, Lavie CJ, Nauman J. Sustained physical activity, not weight loss, associated with improved survival in coronary artery disease. J Am Coll Cardiol 2018; 71: 1094- 1101

14. Xu C, Cao Z. Cardiometabolic diseases, total mortality, and benefits of adherence to a healthy lifestyle: a 13-year prospective UK Biobank study. J Transl Med 2022; 20: 234

15. Kim J, Yang PS, Park BE, et al. Association of light intensity physical activity with mortality in the older population: a nationwide cohort study. Front Cardiovasc Med 2022; 9: 859277

16. Gorcczyca AM, Eaton CB, LaMonte MJ, et al. Change in physical activity and sitting time after myocardial infarction and mortality among postmenopausal women in the women's health initiative-cardiovascular study. J Am Heart Assoc 2017; 6: e005354

17. Wannamethee SG, Shaper AG, Walker M. Physical activity and mortality in older men with diagnosed coronary heart disease. Circulation 2000; 102: 1358- 1363

18. Eckblom O, Ek A, Cider A, et al. Increased physical activity post-myocardial infarction is related to reduced mortality: results from the SWEDENHEART registry. J Am Heart Assoc 2018; 7: e010108

19. Steffen-Batey L, Nichaman MZ, Goff DC Jr, et al. Change in level of physical activity and risk of all-cause mortality or reinfarction: the Corpus Christi Heart Project. Circulation 2000; 102: 2204- 2209

20. Buckley RJR, de Koning IA, Harrison SL, et al. Exercise-based cardiac rehabilitation vs percutaneous coronary intervention for coronary syndrome: impact on morbidity and mortality. Eur Prev Cardiol 2022; 29: 1074- 1080

21. Kang DS, Sung JH, Kim D, et al. Association between exercise habit changes and mortality following a cardiovascular event. Heart 2022; 108: 1945- 1951

22. Mok A, Khaw KT, Luben R, et al. Physical activity trajectories and mortality: population-based cohort study. BMJ 2019; 365: 12323
23. Aggio D, Papachristou E, Papacosta O, et al. Trajectories of physical activity from middle to old age and association with subsequent cardiovascular disease and all-cause mortality. J Epidemiol Comm health 2020; 74: 130- 136
24. Marques Elias RG, Leker ASD, Doa Reis LL, et al. Physical activity, sport practice and cardiovascular risk factors in workers from a public hospital: a trajectory analysis. Front Cardiovasc Med 2021; 8: 740442
25. Barbiellini Amidei C, Trevisan C, Dotto M, et al. Association of physical activity trajectories with major cardiovascular diseases in elderly people, Heart 2022; 108: 360
26. Gonzales-Jaramillo N, Wilhelm M, Arango-Rivas AM, et al. Systematic review of physical activity trajectories with mortality in patients with coronary artery disease. J Am Coll Cardiol 2022; 79: 1690- 1700
27. De Labra C, Guimaraes –Pinheiro C, Maseda A, et al. Effects of physical exercise interventions in older frail adults: a systematic review of randomized controlled trials. BMC Geriatr 2015; 15: 154
28. Haider S, Grabovac I, Dorner TE. Effects of physical activity interventions in frail and prefrail community-dwelling people on frailty status, muscle strength, physical performance and muscle mass-a narrative review. Wiener Klin Wohenschr 2019; 131: 244- 254

29. Izquierdo M, Duque G, Morley JE. Physical activity guidelines for older people: knowledge gaps and future directions. Lancet Healthy Longev 2021; 2: e380-383
30. Grievendonk L, Connell NJ, McCrum C, et al. Impact of aging and exercise on skeletal muscle mitochondrial capacity, energy metabolism, and physical function. Nature Commun 2021; 12: 4773
31. Roberts CK, Little JP, Thyfault JP. Modification of insulin sensitivity and glycemic control by activity and exercise. Med Sci Sports Exerc 2013; 45: 1868- 1877
32. Bird SR, Hawley JA. Update on the effects of physical activity on insulin sensitivity in humans. MBC OpenSport Exerc Med 2016; 2: e000143
33. Colberg SR, Sigal RJ, Yardley JF, et al. Physical activity/exercise and diabetes> A position statement of the American Diabetes Association. Diabetes Care 2016; 39:2065- 2079
34. Egan B, Zierath JR. Exercise metabolism and the molecular regulation of skeletal muscle adaptation. Cell Metab 2013; 17: 162- 164
35. Holloszy JO, Kohurt WM. Regulation of carbohydrate and fat metabolism during and after exercise. Annu Rev Nutr 1996; 16: 121- 138
36. Richter EA, Hargreaves M. Exercise, GLUTA4, and skeletal muscle glucose uptake. Physiol Rev 2013; 93: 993- 1017
37. Hoffman NJ, Parker BL, Chaudhuri R, et al. Global phosphoproteomic analysis of human skeletal muscle reveals a network of exercise-regulated kinases and AMPK substrates. Cell Metab 2015; 22: 922- 935

38. Kraus WF, Houmard JA, Duscha BD, et al. Effects of the amount and intensity of exercise on plasma lipoproteins. N Engl J Med 2002; 347: 1483- 1492
39. Hongeveen RC, Gaubatz JW, Sun W, et al. Small dense low-density lipoprotein-cholesterol concentrations predict risk for coronary heart disease: the atherosclerotic risk in communities (ARIC) study. Atheroscler Thromb Vasc Biol 2014; 34: 1069- 1077
40. Greiwe JS, Holloszy JO, Semenkovish CF. Exercise induces lipoprotein lipase and GLUT-4 protein in muscle independent of adrenergic receptor signaling. J Appl Physiol 2000; 89: 176- 181
41. Duncan GE, Perri MG, Theraque DW, et al. Exercise training without weight loss, increases insulin sensitivity and postheparin plasma lipase activity in previously sedentary adults. Diabetes Care 2003; 26: 557- 562
42. Kazeminasab F, Marandi M, Ghaedi K, et al. Effects of a 4-week aerobic exercise on lipid profile and expression of LXRa in rat liver. Cell J 2017; 19: 45-49
43. McGarrah RW, White PJ. Branched-chain aminoacids in cardiovascular disease. Nature Rev Cardiol 2023; 20: 77- 89
44. Sun H, Olson KC, Cao C, et al. Catabolic defect of branched-chain aminoacids promotes heart failure. Circulation 2016; 133: 2038- 2049
45. Li T, Zhang Z, Kolwicz SC, et al. Defective branched-chain aminoacid catabolism disrupts glucose metabolism and sensitizes the heart to ischemia-reperfusion injury. Cell Metab 2017; 25: 374- 385

46. Tobias DK, Lawler PR, Harada PH, et al. Circulating branched-chain aminoacids and ischemic cardiovascular disease in a prospective cohort of US women. Circ Gnom Precis Med 2018; 11: e002157
47. Wu W, Guo Y, Li M, et al. Exercise enhances the branched-chain aminoacid catabolism and decreases cardiac vulnerability to myocardial ischemic injury. Cells 2022; 11: 1706
48. Chow LS, Gerszten RE, Taylor JM, et al. Exerkines in health, resilience, and disease. Nat Rev Endocrinol 2022; 18: 273- 289
49. Magliulo L, Bondi D, Pini N, et al. The wonder exerkines-novel insights: a critical state-of-the-art review. Mol Cell Biochem 2022; 477: 105- 113
50. Severinsen MCK, Pedersen BK. Muscle-organ crosstalk: the emerging roles of myokines. Endocr Rev 2020; 41: 594- 609
51. Laurens C, Bergouignan A, Moro C. Exercise-related myokines in the control of energy metabolism. Front Physiol 2020; 11: 91
52. Leuchtmann AB, Adak V, Dilbaz S, et al. Therole of skeletal muscle secretome in mediating endurance and resistance training adaptations. Front Physiol 2021; 12: 709807
53. Christensen RH, Lehrskov LL, Wedell-Neergaard AS, et al. Aerobic exercise induces cardiac fat loss and alters cardiac muscle mass trough an Interleukin-6 receptor-dependent mechanism. Cardiac analysis of a double-blind randomized controlled clinical trial in abdominally obese humans. Circulation 2019; 140: 1684- 1686

54. Li A, Dubey S, Varney ML, et al. IL-8 directly enhanced endothelial cell survival, proliferation, and matrix metalloproteinases production and regulated angiogenesis. J Immunol 2003; 170: 3369- 3376
55. Lee DC, Pate RR, Lavie CJ, et al. Leisure-time running reduces all-cause and cardiovascular mortality risk. J Am Coll Cardiol 2014; 64: 472- 481
56. Sesso HD, Stampfer MJ, Rosner B, et al. Systolic and diastolic blood pressure, pulse pressure, and mean arterial pressure as predictors of cardiovascular risk in men. Hypertension 2000; 36: 801- 807
57. Blacher J, Staessen JA, Girerd X, et al. Pulse pressure not mean pressure determines cardiovascular risk in older hypertensive patients. Arch Intern Med 2000; 160: 1085- 1089
58. Donley DA, Fournier SB, Reger BK, et al. Aerobic exercise training reduces arterial stiffness in metabolic syndrome. J Appl Physiol 2014; 116: 1396- 1404
59. Cornelissen VA, Onkelinx S, Goetschalckx K, et al. Exercise-based cardiac rehabilitation improves endothelial function assessed by flow-mediated dilatation but not by pulse amplitude tonometry. Eur J Prev Cardiol 2014; 21: 39- 48
60. Green DJ, Jones H, Thijssen D, et al. Flow-mediated dilation and cardiovascular event prediction. Does nitric oxide matter? Hypertension 2011; 57: 363- 368
61. Ju JS, Jeon SI, Park JY, et al. Autophagy plays a role in skeletal muscle mitochondrial biogenesis in an endurance exercise-trained conditions. J Physiol Sci 2016; 66: 417- 430

62. Lee Y, Kwon I, Jang Y, et al. Potentially signaling pathways in of acute endurance exercise-induced cardiac autophagy and mitophagy and its possible role in cardioprotection. J Physiol Sci 2017; 67: 639- 654
63. Li FH, Li T, Su YM, et al. Cardiac basal autophagic activity and increased exercise capacity. J Physiol Sci 2018; 68: 729- 742
64. Escobar KA, Welch AM, Wells A, et al. Autophagy response to acute high-intensity interval training and moderate continuous training is dissimilar in skeletal muscle and peripheral blood mononuclear cells and influenced by sex. Human Nutr Metab 2021; 23: 200118
65. Chen XK, Zheng C, Siu PMF, et al. Does exercise regulate autophagy in humans? A systemic review and meta-analysis. Autophagy Rep 2023; 2: 1,2190202
66. HallingJF, Pilegaard H. Autophagy-dependent beneficial effects of exercise. Colg Spring Harb Perspect Med 2017; 7: a029777
67. Wu NN, Tian H, Chen P, et al. Physical exercise and selective autophagy: benefit and risk of cardiovascular health. Cells 2019; 8: 1436
68. Wang L, Wang J, Cretoiu D, et a. Exercise-mediated regulation of autophagy in the cardiovascular system. J Sport Health Sci 2020; 9: 203- 210
69. Bravo-San Pedro JM, Kroemer G. Galluzzi L. Autophagy and mitophagy in cardiovascular disease. Circ Res 2017; 120: 1812- 1824
70. Kaludercic N, Maiuri MC, Kaushik S, et al. Comprehensive autophagy evaluation in cardiac disease models. Cardiovasc Res 2020; 116: 483- 504
71. Afshin A, Forouzanfar S, Reitsma MB, et al. Health effects of overweight and obesity in 195 countries over 25 years. N Engl J Med 2017; 377: 13- 27

72. Wormser D, Kaptoge S, Di Angelantonio E, et al. Separate and combined associations of body-mass index and abdominal adiposity with cardiovascular disease: collaborative analysis of 58 prospective studies. Lancet 2011; 377: 1085
73. Kelly T, Yang W, Chen C, et al. Global burden of obesity in 2005 and projections to 2030. Int J Obes 2008; 32: 1431- 1437
74. Powell-Wiley TM, Poirier P, Burke LE, et al. Obesity and cardiovascular disease. A scientific statement from the American Heart Association. Circulation 2021; 143: e984-e1010
75. Gadde KM, Martin CK, Berthound HR, et al. Obesity, pathophysiology and management. J Am Coll Cardiol 2018; 71: 69- 84Effect of 1-year controlled lifestyle intervention on body weight and other risk markers (the healthy lifestyle community program, cohort 2). Obes Facts. 2022; 15: 228- 239
76. Koeder C, Kranz RM, Anand C, et al. Effect of 1-year controlled lifestyle intervention on body weight and other risk markers (the healthy lifestyle community programme, cohort 2). Obes Facts 2022; 15: 228- 239
77. Zhu R, Craciun I, Bernhards-Werge J, et al. Age-and-sex specific effects of long-term lifestyle intervention on body weight and cardiometabolic health markers in adults with prediabetes: results from the diabetes prevention study PREVIW. Dabitologia 2022; 65: 1262- 1277
78. Hammond MM, Zhang Y, Pathiravasan CH, et al. Relations between BMI trajectories and habitual physical activity measured by smart-watch in the electronic cohort of the Framingham heart study: cohort study. MMIR Cadio 2022; 6: e32348

79. Calle EE, Thun MJ, Petrelli JM, et al. Body-mass index and mortality in a prospective cohort of US adults. N Engl J Med 1999; 341: 1097- 1105
80. Hubert HB, Feinleib M, McNamara PM, et al. Obesity as an independent risk factor for cardiovascular disease: a 26-year follow-up of participants in the Framingham heart study. Circulation 1983; 67: 968- 877
81. Manson JF, Willett WC, Stampfer PJ, et al. Body weight and mortality among women. N Engl J Med 1995; 333: 677- 685
82. Folsom AR, Stevens J, Shreiner PJ, et al. Body mass index, waist/hip ratio, and coronary heart incidence in African American and Whites: atherosclerosis risk in communities study investigators. Am J Epidemiolol 1988; 148: 1187- 1194
83. Rogers RP, Bemelmans WJ, Hoogenveen RT, et al. Association of overweight with increased risk of coronary heart disease partly independent of blood pressure and cholesterol levels: a meta-analysis of 21 cohort studies including more than 300,000 persons. Arch Intern Med 2007; 167: 1720- 1728
84. Canoy D, Cairns BJ, Balkwill A, et al. Million women study collaborators. Coronary heart disease incidence in women by waist circumference within categories of body mass index. Eur J Prev Cardiol 2013; 20: 759- 762
85. Zieske AW, Malcom GT, Strong JP. Natural history and risk factors of atherosclerosis in children and youth: the FDAY study. Pediatr Pathol Mol Med 2002; 21: 215- 237
86. Mottilo S, Filion KB, Genest J, et al. The metabolic syndrome and cardiovascular risk: a systematic review and meta-analysis. J Am Coll Cardiol 2010; 56: 1113- 1132

87.Riaz H, Khan MS, Siddiqi TJ, et al. Association between obesity and cardiovascular outcomes: a systematic review and meta-analysis of Mendelian randomized studies. JAMA New Open 2018; 1: e183788101.

88.Di Angelantonio E, Bhupathiraju SN, Wormser D, et al. Body-mass index and all-cause mortality: Individual participant data. Meta-analysis of 239 prospective studies in four continents. Lancet 2016; 388: 776- 786

89.Wu SH, Hui WS, Liu Z, et al. Metabolic syndrome and all-cause mortality: a meta-analysis of prospective cohort studies. Eur J Epidemiol 2010; 25: 375- 384

90.Lin H, Zhang L, Zheng R, et al. The prevalence of metabolic risk and effects of lifestyle intervention for metabolically healthy obesity: a systematic review and meta-analysis: a PRISMA-compliant article. Medicine 2917; 96: e8838

91.Smith GI, Mittendorfer B, Klein S. Metabolically healthy obesity: facts and fantasies. J Clin Invest 2019; 129: 3078- 3989

92.Pattyn N, Cornelisen VA, Toghi Eshghi SR, et al. The effect of exercise on the cardiovascular risk factors constituting the metabolic syndrome. Sports Med 2013; 43: 121- 133

93. Osman C, Smart NA, Marcos D, et al. The effect of exercise training on clinical outcomes in patients with the metabolic syndrome: a systematic review and meta-analysis. Crdiovasc Diabetol 2017; 16: 110

94. Fox CS, Golden SH, Anderson C, et al. Update on prevention of cardiovascular disease in adults with type 2 diabetes mellitus in light of recent evidence. A scientific

statement from the American Heart Association and the American Diabetes Association. Circulation 2015; 132: 691- 718

95. Train WD, Paldanius PM. Diabetes, cardiovascular disease and the microcirculation. Cardiovasc Diabetol 2018; 17: 57

96. Yun JS, Ko SH. Current trends in epidemiology of cardiovascular disease and cardiovascular management in type 2 diabetes. Metab Clin Exper 2021; 123: 154838

97. Tonnies T, Rathmann W, Hoyer A, et al. Quantifying the underestimation of projected global diabetes prevalence by the International Diabetes Federation (IDF) diabetes atlas. BMJ Diab Res Care 2021; 9: e002122

98. Buckley JP, Riddell M, Mellor D, et al. Acute glycemic management before, during and after exercise for cardiac rehabilitation participants with diabetes mellitus: a joint statement of the British and Canadian associations of cardiovascular prevention and rehabilitation and the British association of sport and exercise sciences. Br J Sport Med 2021; 55: 709- 720

99. Holzer R, Schulte-Kome B, Seidler J, et al. Effects of acute resistance endurance exercise with and without whole-body electromyostimulation and endurance exercise on the posprandial glucose regulation in patients with type 2 diabetes mellitus: a randomized crossover study. Nutrients 2021; 13: 4322

100. Mithembu SXH, Mazibuko-Mibeje SE, Ziqubu K, et al. Impact of physical exercise and caloric restriction in patients with type 2 diabetes: skeletal muscle insulin resistance and mitochondrial dysfunction as ideal therapeutic targets. Life Sci 2022; 297: 120467

101. Pinti MV, Fink GK, Hathaway QA, et al. Mitochondrial dysfunction in type 2 diabetes mellitus: an organ-based analysis. Am J Physiol Endocrinol Metab 2019; 316: E268-E285

102. Bhansali S, Bhansali A, Walla R, et al. Alterations in mitochondria oxidative stress and microphagy in subjects with prediabetes and type 2 diabetes mellitus. Front Endocrinol 2017; 8: 347

103. Gonzales CD, Lee MS, Marchetti P, et al. The emerging role of autophagy in the pathophysiology of diabetes mellitus. Autophagy 2011; 7: 2- 11

104. Kruse R, Vind BF, Petersson SJ, et al. Markers of autophagy are adapted to hyperglycemia in skeletal muscle in type 2 diabetes. Diabetologia 2015; 58: 2067- 2095

105. Etehad D, Emdin CA, Kiran A, et al. Blood pressure lowering for prevention of cardiovascular disease and death: a systematic review and meta-analysis. Lancet 2016; 387: 957- 967

106. Brunstrom M, Carlberg B. Association of blood pressure lowering with mortality and cardiovascular disease across blood pressure levels: a systematic review and meta-analysis. JAMA Intern Med 2018; 178: 28- 36

107. Luo D, Cheng Y, Zhang H, et al. Association between high blood pressure and long cardiovascular events in young adults: a systematic review and meta-analysis. BMJ Open Access 2020; 370: m32231

108. The Blood Pressure Lowering Treatment Trialists Collaboration. Pharmacological blood pressure lowering for primary and secondary prevention of cardiovascular

disease across different levels of blood pressure: an individual participant- level data meta-analysis. Lancet 2021; 397: 1625- 1636

109. Flint AC, Conell C, Ren X, et al. Effect of systolic and diastolic blood pressure on cardiovascular outcomes. N Engl J Med 2019; 381: 243- 251

110. Fu Y, Feng Q, Wei Y, et al. Meta-analysis of the effect of aerobic training on blood pressure in hypertensive patients. Comp Math Methods Med 2022; 2022: 9281661

1111. Saco-Ledo G, Valenzuela PL, Ruilope LM, et al. Physical exercise in resistant hypertension: a systematic review and meta-analysis of randomized controlled trials. Front Cardiovasc Med 2022; 9: 893811

112. Wen H, Wang L. Reducing effect of aerobic exercise on blood pressure of essential hypertensive patients: a meta-analysis. Medicine 2017; 96: e6150

113. Arciero PJ, Ives SJ, Mohr AE, et al. Morning exercise reduces abdominal fat and blood pressure in women; evening exercise increases muscular performance in women and lowers blood pressure in men. Front Physiol 2022; 13: 893783

114. Dimeo F, Pagonas N, Seibert F, eta al. Aerobic exercise reduces blood pressure in resistant hypertension. Hypertension 2012; 60: 653- 658

115. Schmitt EE, McNair BD, Olson SM, et al. Mechanisms of exercise-induced cardiac remodeling differ between young and aged hearts. Exerc Sport Sci Rev 2022; 50: 137- 144

116. Weiner RB, Baggish AL. Exercise-induced cardiac remodeling. Prog Cardiovas Dis 2013; 54: 380- 386

117. Boyle AJ, Shih H, Hwang J, et al. Cardiomyopathy of aging in the mammalian heart is characterized by myocardial hypertrophy, fibrosis and predisposition towards cardiomyocyte apoptosis and autophagy. Exp Gerontol 2011; 46: 549- 559

118. Cheng S, Xanthakis V, Sullivan LM, et al. Correlates of echocardiographic indices of cardiac remodeling over the adult life course: longitudinal observations from the Framingham Heart Study. Circulation 2010; 122: 570 – 578

119. Dazoti Debessa CR, Msiano Mifrino LB, Rodrigues deSouza R. Age related changes of the collagen network of the human heart. Mech Ageing Dev 2001; 122: 1049- 1058

120. Capasso JM, Palackal T, Olivetti G, et al. Severe myocardial dysfunction induced by ventricular remodeling in aging rat hearts. Am j Physiol 1990; 259 (4 Part 2): H1086- H1096

121. Archley AF Jr, Douglas PS. Left ventricular hypertrophy in athletes: morphological features and clinical correlates. Cardiol Clin 2007' 25: 371- 382

122. Kemi CJ, Haram PM, Loennechen JP, et al. Moderate vs high exercise intensity: differential effects on aerobic fitness, cardiomyocyte contractility, and endothelial function. Cardiovasc Res 2005; 67: 161- 172

123. Hwang CL, Too JK, Kim HK, et al. Novel all-extremity high-intensity interval training improves aerobic fitness, cardiac function and insulin resistance in healthy older adults. Exp Gerontol 2016; 82: 112- 119

124. Vega RB, Konhilas JP, Kelly DP, et al. Molecular mechanisms underlying cardiac adaptations to exercise. Cell Metab 2017; 25: 1012- 1026

125. Arem H, Moore SC, Patel A, et al. Leisure time physical activity and mortality: a detailed pooled analysis of the dose-response relationship. JAMA Intern Med 2015; 175: 959- 967

126. Tipton CM. The history of "exercise medicine" in ancient civilizations. Adv Physiol Educ 2014; 38: 109- 117

127. Castelletti S, D'Ascenzi F, Papadakis M. Sports cardiology in Europe from ancient to Greek-Roman era to the present. Eur Heart J 2022; 43: 2542- 2544

128. Nesti L, Pugliese NR, Sciuto P, et al. Type 2 diabetes and reduced exercise tolerance: a review of the literature through an integrated physiologic approach. Cardiovasc Diabetol 2020; 19: 134

129, Pugliese NR, De Biase N, Gargani L, et al. Predicting the transition to and progression of heart failure with preserved ejection fraction: a weighted risk score using bio-humoral cardiopulmonary and echocardiographic stress testing. Eur Prev Cardiol 2021; 28: 1650- 1661

130. Nesti L, Pugliese NR, Sciuto P, et al. Mechanisms of reduced peak oxygen consumption in subjects with uncomplicated type 2 diabetes. Cardiovasc Diabetol 2021; 120: 124

131. Pugliese NR, De Biase N, Balletti A, et al. Characterization of hemodynamic and metabolic abnormalities in the heart failure spectrum: the role of combined

cardiopulmonary and exercise echocardiography stress test. Minerva Cardiol Angiol 2022; 70: 370- 3784

132. Giallauria F, Strscluglio T, Cuomo G, et al. Exercise training: the holistic approach in cardiovascular prevention. High Blood Press Cardiovasc Prev 2021; 28: 561- 577

Chapter Three

The Effects of Physical Activity on Sleep Quality and Wellbeing

Introduction

Regular PA has pluripotential CV and body effects by reducing the incidence of CVD, CHD, T2DM, hypertension, and increasing body strength and mobility [1]. In addition, recent studies suggest that PA exerts beneficial effects on the onset, duration, and quality of sleep, which very important for a healthy physical and mental wellbeing [2-4]. In addition, PA plays an important role in smoothing out fragmented and disturbed sleep in older people, restores their mental and physical condition and prevents health problems [5-7]. In this regard, PA is considered a n effective non-pharmacological approach in improving sleep quality and is complementary to patients with sleep problems [8]. The first ever study on the effects of exercise on sleep quality was done by Backeland and Lasky in 10 physically fit students, and showed that afternoon exercise resulted in significant increase in slow wave sleep (SWS) stages 3 and 4 (deep sleep) compared to non-exercise [9]. In contrast, the effects of evening exercise were smaller and fell between afternoon exercise and non-exercise. With respect to the levels of PA on sleep, it has been by Koohsari et al [10], in 683 Japanese subjects ages 40-64 years, that sleep length and sleep quality increased from sedentary behavior to light PA, to moderate-vigorous PA in women, but not in men. Another study by Wendt, et al [11], in 1993 subjects mean age 22.6 years, using an accelerometer showed that morning exercise conferred the best results regarding sleep quality, whereas evening exercise had the opposite effects. However, any type of PA including Tai Chi confers significant effects on sleep improvement in older adults with insomnia [12]. For the effect of PA on sleep duration and quality the English literature was searched between 2017 and 2023 and 36 pertinent papers were selected. The results from these papers together wirh collateral literature will be discussed.

Beneficial Effects of Physical Activity on Sleep Quality

Many studies and reviews have demonstrated beneficial effects of PA on sleep and sleep quality [13-21]. These studies are summarized in Table 1 and they will be , briefly, discussed here. Dolezal et al [13], analyzed the effects of different types and levels of exercise on sleep and sleep quality in a review of 34 studies involving 506,649 subjects ages 18-79 years. The subjects included in this review had different types of sleep problems and were involved in different types and durations of PA. Overall, the PA improved their sleep, its duration and quality. The study by Ezati et al [14], was designed to evaluate the effects of of regular aerobic exercise on sleep quality and fatigue in 67 female students ages 18-26 years. The students were subjected to 1 hr of aerobic exercise of mild to moderate intensity three times/week for 8 weeks. The exercise resulted in significant improvement in sleep duration and quality compared to a control group ($p < 001$), respectively. The study by Thomas et al [15], evaluated the effects of early evening high-intensity exercise on sleep duration in 8 endurance runners mean age 27.8 ± 8.9 years. The participants were subjected 3.5 hours before sleep to 1.0 hour of high intensity internal running at 90% VO_{2peak} with 5 min rest, then 1 hour of low-intensity running at 45% VO_{2peak} and then to rest (control). High-intensity exercise was associated with sleep duration of 477.4 ± 17.7 min ($p = 0.022$), whereas low-intensity exercise resulted in sleep duration of 479.6 ± 15.6 min ($p = 0.006$), compared to control group of sleep duration of 462.9 ± 19 min. In addition, awake time was shorter with high and low-intensity exercise by 31.8 ± 18.5 min, ($p = 0.047$), and by 30.4 ± 15.7 min ($p = 0.008$) compared to 46.6 ± 20 min for the control group. In this study, the sleep duration was evaluated objectively with polysomnography and wristwatch actigraphy. This small study showed that late evening exercise does not disturb sleep duration. The study by Park and Suh [16], evaluated the amount of PA and shift work on the quality of sleep in 185,958 full time workers mean age 40 years. The amount of PA was evaluated in METs-min/week. A regression analysis showed that increased PA of 600-9000 METs-min/week was associated with improved sleep quality compared to a sedentary group. In men and women day workers, sleep quality improved with the level of PA, OR 0.825 (95% CI 0.737-0.924) for women and OR 0.777 (95% CI 0.735-0.821) for PA 3000 to < 6000 METs-min/week ($p < 0.001$). For Pa 6000 to < 9000 METs-min/week the ORs were 1.061 (95% CI 0;835-1.348, p< 0.627)) for women and 0.759 (95% CI 0.672 -0.856, p < 001) for men. However, the results were less favorable between exercise and quality of sleep for shift workers of both sexes. Much higher levels of PA of 9000 to < 12000 METs-min/week were not associated with improved sleep quality for either day work or shift work for men and women. In a review and meta-analysis Xie et al [17], analyzed the effects of exercise on sleep quality and insomnia in 22 randomized trials involving 1806 subjects ages 16-76 with different types and durations of exercise using the Pittsburg Sleep Quality Index (PSQI) and Insomnia Severity Index (ISI). The analysis of results showed that exercise improved significantly, the quality of sleep in adults compared to controls with lower PSQI, mean difference (MD) – 2.19 (95% CI – 2.96 to – 1.41), and ISI MD – 1.52 (95% CI - 2.63 to – 0.41). Interestingly, short-term interventions (≤ 3 monts) had significantly greater reduction in sleep disturbances than long-term interventions (> 3 months). In addition, exercise besides improving nighttime sleep and insomnia, it also improved daytime sleepiness. In a large study Huang et al [18], evaluated the effects of different levels of PA on sleep and on the risk of all-cause and CVD and cancer mortality in 380,055 participants from the UK Biobank mean age 55.9 ± 8.1 years. They divided the participants into high, medium, low and no moderate-to- vigorous PA (MVPA). After 11.1 years of follow-up, the group with the no MVPA had the highest risk of all-cause and CVD mortality, HR 1.57 (95% CI 1.35-1.82), and 1.67 (95% CI 1.27-2.19), respectively compared to high intensity PA group. This study showed a synergistic effect of PA on good sleep and the prevention of CVD and all-cause mortality. In a review and meta-analysis, Fank et al [19] analyzed the effects of exercise from 20 studies involving 5066 older subjects. The participants were divided into an exercise and control group and the effects of exercise on sleep were assessed subjectively and objectively. The exercise group compared to control group showed subjective improvement in the PSQI score, standardized mean difference (SMD) – 0.68 (95% CI – 0.82 to – 0.55. p < 0.001), subjective sleep quality, SMD – 0.77 (95% CI – 1.20 to – 0.33, p < 0.001), sleep latency, SMD – 0,72 (95% CI – 1.11 to – 0.33, p < 0.001), and sleep tendency SMD – 0.32 (95% CI – 0.52 to – 0.11, p < 0.001), habitual sleep efficiency, SMD -0.24 (95% CI – 0.45 to – 0.03, p = 0.020), sleep disturbance, SMD – 0.30 (95% CI – 0.59 to -0.00, p = 0.05), sleep medication, SMD – 0.45 (95% CI – 0.73 to – 0.18, p = 0.001), sleep dysfunction, SMD – 0.41 (95% CI – 0.78 to – 0. 04, p = 0.03) and no effect on day time sleepiness. Objectively, exercise improved only sleep onset latency SMD – 0.86 (95% CI – 1.48 to – 0.24, p = 0.007) and had no effect on total sleep time and sleep efficiency. In specially designed study, Mochon-Beguigui et al

[20], evaluated the effects of sedentariness, PA levels, and physical fitness on sleep quality in 74 sedentary middle age adults (53.7 ± 5.1 years). PA and objective sleep parameters were measured by accelerometry and subjective parameters by the PSQI. Reduced levels of sedentariness, greater VO_{2max} and muscular strength were associated with sleep improvement and sleep quality and quantity ($p \leq 0.05$). In a review and meta-analysis, Zhao et al [21] analyzed the effects of different levels of PA on sleep quality in 3311 subjects ages 14-52 years. The 288 children mean age 4.3i ± 0.8 years this review, were removed from the analysis of results. Sleep quality was evaluated by the PSQUI, the Athens insomnia scale (AIS), the wristband sleep watch, the International Physical Activity Questionnaire (IPAQ), and the German Physical Activity Exercise and Sports Questionnaire (BSA-F). The analysis of results showed that sleep quality was improved in middle-aged and elderly persons, mean difference (MD), 1.98, $p = 0.03$, but not in young people, MD 1..32 ($p = 0.11$). Moderate-intensity PA improved quality of sleep, but high-intensity PA had no obvious effect on sleep quality.

No Association of Physical Activity and Sedentary Behavior on Sleep Quality

Although the great majority of studies shows a positive effect on sleep and sleep quality, there are a few studies that have not shown a definite improvement with PA on sleep quality [22,23]. In one study by Youngstedt et al [22] of 102 subjects, 31 students mean age 22.9 ± 2.8 years and 71adults ages 18-75 years. The effect of PA activity on sleep was assessed by actigraphy and sleep diaries. There was no significant effect of PA on sleep. In the other study, Kahn et al [23], evaluated the effects of evening PA on sleep quality in 12,638 subjects mean age 40.1 ± 10.1 years by Polar wearable devices for 14 consecutive days. Moderate to near maximal exercise performed during 3 hours before sleep showed that sleep efficiency was not significantly associated with sleep efficiency. This study demonstrated that exercise performed before sleep was not associated with objective and suggestive sleep efficiency and suggests that exercise performed a few hours before sleep does not affect sleep and should not be discouraged. In contrast other investigators including the American Academy of Sleep medicine, discourage evening exercise that the excitement from exercise could delay the onset of sleep [24,25]. These statements have been refuted by many other studies, which in addition have shown that the adverse cardiovascular and sleep effects of inactivity are reversed in people who switch from inactivity to regular PA [26-30].

Pathophysiology of Exercise on Sleep

Adequate sleep and exercise are biological necessities due to their effects on wellbeing and prevention of chronic adverse health effects [31,32]. The pathophysiology of exercise on sleep is complex and not well understood at preset. Exercise induces several factors, such as stimulation of the central nervous system (CNS), induction of fatigue, temporary increase in body temperature, increase in heart rate variability (HRV), stimulation of hormonal factors, decrease in blood glucose, the brain derived neurogenic factor, and the insulin-like growth factor-1 (IGF-1). These changes induced by exercise are depicted in Figure 1 and are briefly, discussed here. **1) CNS effect:** Sleep is mainly consisted of two phases such as the rapid eye movement (REM) sleep, and no rapid eye movement (NREM) sleep or slow wave sleep (SWS), which is consisted of 4 stages (N1-N4). Several studies have shown that both acute and chronic exercise affect the REM and NREM sleep by prolonging the NREM and shortening the

REM sleep [33]. Chronic exercise improves autonomic nervous system balance by reducing sympathetic nerve activity and increasing parasympathetic nerve activity with improvement on NREM sleep, which is the deep sleep [34]. **2) Body temperature:** The body by Horne and Staff [35], showed that light exercise at 40% VO_{2max} for 160 min did not affect the body temperature, increased REM and NREM sleep and decreased sleep onset time. The other study by Flausino et al [36], showed that exercise did not affect the body temperature and improved REM sleep. The sight increase in body temperature with exercise is dissipated [37]. quickly through vasodilation and sweating and does not affect sleep. **3) Heart Rate Variability:** Short and long-term exercise is associated with increase in HR and HRV, eventually increases vagal modulation and increase in HRV and NREM sleep [38]. Also, during sleep there are significant differences in the parasympathetic modulation in young than middle-age persons. Young people exhibit higher parasympathetic activity during sleep, which helps them sleep better than older people [39]. **Hormonal Effects of Exercise: a) Growth Hormone:** Moderate to high intensity exercise increases growth hormone (GH) secretion during sleep and increases the slow wave sleep (SWS) in contrast to inactivity [40], The GH release occurs and could be a correlation between GH and SWS, since GH-releasing factor injections in humans is associated with decreased wakefulness and increased SWS [42]. Also, age-related decrease in GH release could be associated with the decreased sleep of older subjects. **2). b) Melatonin:** Melatonin is a key hormone that regulates circadian rhythm and sleep and is increased with exercise [43,44]. **C) Cortisol:** Regarding the release of cortisol with exercise, there is some controversy with some studies showing a decrease with exercise [43], and other showing an increase [45]. However, cortisol has a diurnal variation with increased levels in the morning and decreased levels in the evening. This is important because cortisol suppresses melatonin release and this could disturb sleep. **5) Brain-Derived Neurotrophic Factor:** The brain-derived neurotrophic factor (BDNF) is a key molecule synthesized by the brain neurons and plays a significant role in the brain functions and could play a role in sleep regulation with exercise [46,47], since it has been demonstrated that sleep deprivation in normal subjects has been associated with low levels of BDNF [48]. However, more work is needed to clarify the role of BDNF on sleep. **6) Insulin-like growth hormone -1 (IGH-1).** The release of IGH-1 is stimulated by GH which is increased with exercise and emerging evidence suggests a possible role of IGH-1 on brain plasticity and sleep [49]. Previous studies have shown that intracerebral injections of IGH-1 were associated with an increase in NREM and REM sleep [50].

Discussion

Sleep and exercise play a vital role in maintaining human health and wellbeing, and many studies have demonstrated the positive effect of exercise on sleep duration and quality [13-21]. The 17th century philosophers Descartes and Locke were fascinated with role of sleep, with Descartes believing that the sleeping brain continues to think, and Locke believing that the sleeping brain was inactive and by extension of limited purpose [51]. However, later electroengephalographic studies challenged this notion and demonstrated that the brain is active during sleep [52]. A good sleep is crucial for healthy wellbeing and mental health and could enhance cognition and the ability to engage in several activities [51]. Regular exercise has been shown to be a non-pharmacological intervention that improves sleep and sleep quality [6,13-21,53]. The potential mechanisms by which exercise improves sleep and sleep quality are several and are depicted in figure 1. The Physical Activity Guideline Advisory Committee and the American College of Sports Medicine recommend a multi-component exercise combining endurance, strength, balance and flexibility training to improve sleep, physical health, and wellbeing [54]. Other studies have also shown that multi-component exercise may directly or indirectly affect sleep quality and mental function [55-57]. Other types of exercise like Tai Chi, Pilates, or Yoga, may also enhance sleep and sleep quality [58-60]. Regarding sleep duration, adults need between 7-8 hours/night [61-63]. In a recent study, sleep duration of ≤ 5 hours/night was associated with increased incidence of multimorbidity, Hr 1.30 (95% CI 1.12-1.50, $p < 0.001$), whereas sleep duration ≥ 9 hour/night was not [64]. The need for sleep is slightly deceased with the advancement of age as was demonstrated in a recent study after 36 years of follow-up [65]. Regarding the overall effects of exercise, this review has shown that exercise is beneficial for body and mind wellbeing through its multipotential beneficial cardiovascular and sleep effects.

Conclusion: This brief review of the literature has demonstrated that physical activity of any kind and any level, improves general health and sleep duration and quality. A good sleep is necessary for the maintenance of body and mental wellbeing and it should be encouraged for people of all ages. A normal sleep duration of 7-8 hours/night is recommended by the American College of Sports Medicine and WHO, in order to be able to perform successfully our daily activities. In contrast, sleep deprivation (≤ 5 hours/night) has been associated with adverse cardiovascular and mental effects including death. In this respect, exercise serves as a non-pharmacologic therapy and can be complimentary to medical therapy. Therefore, any type of exercise, light to moderate to vigorous performed any time during the day is very helpful for the maintenance of good health.

Figure Legend

Figure 1. This figure depicts the various factors induced by exercise, which mediate the effects of exercise on the duration and quality of sleep.

References

1. Chrysant SG, Chrysant GS. Association of physical activity and trajectories of physical activity with cardiovascular disease. Expert Rev Cardiovasc Ther 2023; 21: 87- 96
2. Li J, Cao D, Huang Y, et al. Sleep duration and health outcomes: an umbrella review. Sleep Breath 2022; 26: 1479- 1501
3. Yin J, Jin X, Shan Z, et al. Relationship of sleep duration and all-cause mortality and cardiovascular events: a systematic review and dose-response meta-analysis of prospective cohort studies. J Am Heart Assoc 2017; 6: e005947
4. Jike M, Itani O, Watanabe N, et al. Long sleep duration and health outcomes: a systematic review, meta-analysis and meta-regression. Sleep Med Rev 2018; 39: 25- 36
5. Irwin MR. Why sleep is important for health: a psychosoneuroimmunology perspective. Annu Rev Psychol 2015; 66: 143- 172
6. Wang F, Boros S. The effect of physical activity on sleep quality: a systematic review. Eur J Physiother 2021; 23: 11- 18

7. Le Cornu Q, Chen M, van Hees V, et al. Association of physical activity, sedentary behaviour, and daylight exposure with sleep in an ageing population: findings from the Whitehall accelerometer sub-study. Int J Behav Nutr Phys Act 2022; 19: 144

8. Yang PY, Ho KH, Chen HC, et al. Exercise training improves sleep quality in middle-aged and older adults with sleep problems: a systematic review. J Physiother 2012; 58: 157- 163

9. Backeland F, Lasky R. Exercise and sleep quality patterns in college athletes. Percept Mot Skills 1966; 23: 1203- 1207

10. Koohsari MJ, Yasunnaga A, McCormack GR, et al. Sedentary behaviour and sleep quality. Sci Rep 2023; 13: 1180

11. Wendt A, da Silva ICM, Goncalves H, et al. Short-term effects of physical activity of sleep health: a population-based study using accelerometry. J Sport Health Sci 2022; 11: 630- 638

12. Su PM, Yu AP, Tam BT, et al. Effects of Tai Chi exercise on sleep in older adults with insomnia: a randomized clinical trial. JAMS Open 2021; 4: e2037199

13. Dolezal BA, Neufeld EV, Boland DM, et al. Interrelationship between sleep and exercise: a systematic review. Adv Prev Med 2017; 2017: 1364387

14. Ezati M, Keshavarz M, Amirkhanzadeh Z, et al. The effect of regular aerobic exercise on sleep quality and fatigue among female student dormitory residents. BMC Sports Sci Med Rehabbil 2020; 12: 44

15. Thomas C, Jones H, Whitworth-Turner C, et al. High-intensity exercise in the evening does not disrupt sleep in endurance runners. Eur J Appl Physiol 2020; 120: 359- 368
16. Park H, Suh B. Association between sleep quality and physical activity according to gender and shift work. J Sleep Res 2020; 29: e12924
17. Xie Y, Liu S, Chen XJ, et al. Effects of exercise on sleep quality and insomnia in adults: a systematic review and meta-analysis of randomized control trials. Front Psychiatry 2021; 12: 664499
18. Huang BH, Duncan MJ, Cistulli PA, et al. Sleep and physical activity in relation to all-cause, cardiovascular disease and cancer mortality risk. Br J Sports Med 2022; 56: 718- 724
19. Fank F, da Silva Pereira F, dos Santos L, et al. Effects of exercise on sleep in older adults: an overview of systemic reviews and meta-analyses. J Aging Phys Act 2022; 30: 1101- 1117
20. Mochon-Beguigui S, Carneiro-Barrera A, Castillo M, et al. Role of physical activity and fitness on sleep in sedentary middle-aged adults: the FIT-AGEING study. Sci Rep 2023; 11: 539
21. Zhao H, Lu C, Yi C. Physical activity and sleep quality association in different populations: a meta-analysis. Int J Envirom Res Public Health 2023; 20: 1864
22. Youngsteadt S, Perlis ML, O'Brien PM, et al. No association of sleep with total daily physical activity and normal sleepers. Physiol Behav 2003; 78: 395- 401

23. Kahn M, Korhonen T, Leinonen L, et al. Is it time we stop discouraging evening physical activity? New real-world evidence from 150,000 nights. Front Public Health 2021; 9: 772376

24. Oda S, Shirakawa K. Sleep onset is disrupted following pre-sleep exercise that causes large physiological excitement at bedtime. Eur J Appl Physiol 2014; 114: 1789- 1799

25. American Sleep Association, 2021 available at www,aasmnet.org

26. Seol J, Abe T, Fujii Y, et al. Effect of sedentary behaviour and physical activity on sleep quality in older people: a cross-sectional study. Nurs Health Sci 2020; 22: 64- 71

27. Jeong SH, Jang BN, Kim SH, et al. Association between sedentary time and sleep quality based on the Pittsburg Sleep Quality Index among South Korean adults. BMC Publ Health 2021; 21: 2290

28. You Y, Chen Y, Fanf W, et al. The association between sedentary behavior, exercise, and sleep disturbance: a mediation analysis of inflammatory biomarkers. Front Immunol 2023; 13: 1080782

29. Koohsari MJ, Yasuaga A, McCormack GR, et al. Sedentary behaviour and sleep quality. Sci Rep 2023; 13: 1180

30. Chrysant SG, Chrysant GS. The cardiovascular consequences of excess sitting time. J Clin Hypertens 2015; 17: 528- 531

31. Ramar K, Malhorta PK, Carden KA, et al. Sleep is essential to health: an American Academy of Sleep Medicine position statement. J Clin Sleep Med 2021; 17: 10

32. Chrysant SG, Chrysant GS. Association of physical activity and trajectories of physical activity with cardiovascular disease. Expert Rev Cardiovasc Ther 2023; 21: 87- 96
33. Uchida S, Shioda K, Morita Y, et al. Exercise effects on sleep physiology. Front Neurol 2012; 3: 49
34. Locket E. 2020. Sleep stages, available at https://www.healthline.com/health/health-sleep/stages-of-sleep
35. Home JA, Staff LHE. Exercise and sleep: body-heating effects. Sleep 1983; 6: 36- 46
36. Flausino NH, Da Silva Prado MJ, de Queiroz SS, et al. Physical exercise performed before bedtime improves the sleep pattern in healthy young good sleepers. Pathophysiology 2012; 49: 186-
37. Michael S, Graham KS, Davis GM. Cardiac autonomic responses during exercise and post-exercise recovery using heart rate variability and systolic time intervals- a review. Front Physiol 2017; 8: 301
38. Catal AM, Chacon-Mikahil MRT, Martinelli FS, et al. Effects of aerobic exercise training on heart rate variability during wakefulness and sleep and cardiorespiratory responses of young and middle-age healthy men. Braz J Med Biol Res 2002; 35: 741- 752
39. Kanaley JA, Weltman KY, Veldhuis JD, et al. Human growth hormone response to repeated bouts of aerobic exercise. Clin Neurophysiol 1997; 83: 1756- 1761
40. Van Cauter E, Plat L. Physiology of growth hormone secretion during sleep. J Pediatr 1996; 128(Part 2): S32-S37

41. Torsvail L, Akerstedt T, Lindbeck G. Effects of deep stages and EEG power density of different degrees of exercise in fit subjects. Electroencephalogr Clin Neurophysiol 1984; 57: 347- 353

42. Adamson L, Hunter WM, Ogunremi OO, et al. Growth hormone increase during sleep after daytime exercise. J Endocrinol 1974; 62: 473- 478

43. Harinath K, Malhotra AS, Pal K, et al. Effects of Hatha yoga and Omkar meditation on cardiorespiratory performance, physiologic profile, and melatonin secretion. J Altern Complement Med 2001; 10: 261- 268

44. Lee H, Kim S, Kim D, et al. Effects of exercise with and without light exposure on sleep quality and hormone responses. J Exerc Nutr Biochem 2014; 18: 293- 299

45. Monteleone P, Fuschino A, Nolfe G, et al. Temporal relationship between melatonin and cortisol responses to nighttime physical stress in humans. Psychoendocrinol 1992; 17: 81- 86

46. Miranda M, Facundo Morici J, Belen Zanoni M, et al. Brain-derived neurotrophic factor: a key molecule for memory in healthy and pathologic brain. Front Cellular Neurosci 2019; 13: 363

47. Jimenez-Maldonado A, Renteria I, Garcia-Suarez PC, et al. The impact of high-intensity interval training on brain-derived neurotrophic factor in brain: a mini review. Front Neurosci 2016; 12: 839

48. Eckert A, Karen S, Beck J, et al. The link between sleep, stress, and BDNF. Eur Psychiatry 2017; 41: 839

49. Chennaoui M, Leger D, Gomez-Merino D. Sleepand the GH/IGF-1 axis: consequences and countermeasures of sleep loss/disorders. Sleep Med Rev 2020; 49: 101223

50. Obal F, Jr, Kapas L, Bodosi B, et al. Changes in sleep response to intracerebral injection of insulin-like growth factor-1 (IGF-1) in the rat. Sleep Res Online 1998; 1: 87- 91

51. Fink AM, Bronas UG, Galik MW. Autonomic regulation during sleep and wakefulness: a review with implications for defining the pathophysiology of neurological disorders. Clin Auton Res 2018; 28: 509- 518

52. Aserinsky E, Kleitman. Regularly occurring periods of eye motility, and concomitant phenomena during sleep. Science 1953; 118: 273- 274

53. Banno M, Harada Y, Taniguchi M, et al. Exercise can improve sleep quality: a systematic review and meta-analysis. Peer J 2018; 6: e5172

54. Piercy KL, Trolano RP, Ballard RM, et al. The physical activity guidelines for Americans. JAMA 2018; 320: 2020- 2028

55. Timmons JF, Minnock D, Hone M, et al. Comparison of time-matched aerobic, resistance, or concurrent exercise training in older adults. Scand J Med Sci Sports 2018; 28: 2272- 2283

56. Larkey L, Jahnke R, Etnier J, et al. Meditative movement as a category of exercise. J Phys Act Health 2009; 6: 230- 238

57. Low H, Haddock G, Mulligan LD, et al. Does exercise improve sleep for adults with insomnia? A systematic review with quality appraisal. Clin Physiol Rev 2019; 68: 1- 12

58. Su PM, Yu AP, Tam BT, et al. Effects of Tai Chi or exercise on sleep in older adults with insomnia. A randomized clinical trial. JAMA Open 2021; 4: e2037199

59. Chen Z, Ye X, Shen Z, et al. Effects of Pilates on sleep quality. A systematic review and meta-analysis of randomized controlled trials. Front Neurol 2020; 11: 168

60. Baklouti S, Fekih-Romhane F, Guelmani N, et al. The effect of web-based yoga on physiological distress and sleep quality in older adults: a randomized controlled trial. Compl Ther Clin Pract 2023; 50: 101715

61. Bull FC, Al-Ansari SS, Biddle S, et al. World Health Organization 2020 guidelines on physical activity and sedentary behaviour. Br J Sports Med 2020; 54: 1451-1462

62. Chaput JP, Dutil C, Featherstone R, et al. Sleep duration and health in adults: an overview of systematic reviews. Appl Physiol Nutr Metab 2020; 45: 5218- 5231

63. Watson NF, Badr MS, Belanky G, et al. Recommended amount of sleep for a healthy adult: a Joint Statement of the American Academy of Sleep Medicine and Sleep Research Society. J Clin Sleep Med 2015; 11: 6

64. Sabia S, Dugravot A, Leger D, et al. Association of sleep duration at age 50, 60, and 70 years with the risk of multimorbidity in the UK: a 25-year follow-up of the Whitehall II cohort study. PloS Med 2022; 19(10): e1004109

65. Hublin C, Haasio L, Kaprio J. Changes in self-reported sleep duration with age- a 36-year longitudinal study of Finnish adults. BMC Public Health 2020; 20: 1373

Publisher: Eliva Press Global Ltd

Email: info@elivapress.com